Traditional Chinese Medicine: Esthetician's Guide

Dr. Michelle O'Shaughnessy, D.O.M., C.I.D.E.S.C.O. Diplomate

Traditional Chinese Medicine: Esthetician's Guide

ISBN: 978-1-932633-31-3

Editorial

Book Editor:	Angela C. Kozlowski
Copy Editor:	Timothy Lockman
Indexer:	Joy Dean Lee
Proofreader:	Emily S. Keats
Designer:	Hon Bannapradist

Administration

Publisher:	Marian S. Raney
Book Manager:	Marie Kuta
Book Coordinator and Web Support:	Anita Singh

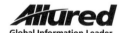

Global Information Leader

Allured Publishing Corporation
336 Gundersen Drive, Carol Stream, IL 60188 USA
Tel: 630-653-2155   Fax: 630-653-2192
E-mail: books@allured.com

Table of Contents

About the Author

Michelle O'Shaughnessy was born in Florida. During her formative years, she lived in Bogota, Colombia, where she became fluent in Spanish. She began her academia in Florida, then continued at the Sorbonne Universite in Paris, where she had her first facial and fell in love with skin care. She earned her Bachelors degree from the University of Central Florida in anthropology and Latin American studies. She is now a Doctor of Oriental Medicine who graduated cum laude with a Masters in Oriental Medicine from the Florida College of Integrative Medicine in Orlando, Florida. Additionally, she has received several advanced certifications in acupuncture facelifts and cosmetic acupuncture.

O'Shaughnessy is the proud owner of an Aesthetic Acupuncture Clinic in Orlando. Her clinic specializes in acupuncture facelifts and is among the first to incorporate facials, Chinese herbs, acupuncture and skin care to help improve skin care concerns including acne, rosacea, anti-aging, rashes, psoriasis as well as women's general health. In addition to owning her clinic, she is also an Account Executive for "Chi Infusion," a skincare line based on Chinese herbs.

O'Shaughnessy has a strong passion for studying traditional Chinese medicine and herbal remedies for the skin. She completed an internship in China at the "Chinese PLA General Hospital," the largest military hospital in Beijing. She is a board member of the Guatemala Acupuncture and Medical Aid Project (G.U.A.M.A.P.), which is a non-profit organization that teaches acupuncture to the Mayan Indians in the Peten region of Guatemala.

Michelle has been an esthetician for over twelve years. She has worked for Sothys-USA as a national trainer as well as for Babor as an account executive.

Acknowledgment

This book would not have been possible without the support of my incredible husband Philip and my two wonderful sons, Robert and John. The three of them encouraged me during my C.I.D.E.S.C.O. examination process and then through three years of graduate school. Philip supported me and took care of the kids while I did an internship in China and supported me financially so I could concentrate on writing this book. He worked diligently beside me on the soup chapter and was able to bring his extensive culinary experience and knowledge as a professional chef to the soup section of this book. Without his input, the soups wouldn't be so delicious.

The other person I want to acknowledge is my mother. She is the person that I admire and try to emulate in my life. She got her Masters and PhD in Nutrition. While I was in high school, she experimented on her three daughters with different health concoctions and taught the benefits of alternative health and nutrition that we have practiced our entire lives. She was also the person who read every chapter as it was written, gave me her feedback and helped me with all my rewrites to make sure that my ideas flowed smoothly.

I also want to acknowledge my brilliant professors at the Florida College of Integrative Medicine (FCIM), in Orlando, Florida. My teachers taught me the benefits and effectiveness of this amazing medical discipline. All who teach at FCIM are passionate about mentoring their students to be devoted to their patients' health. Furthermore, they guided me in perfecting my herbal formulations and skin treatments.

THANK YOU!

Preface

Why do we need a book on traditional Chinese medicine for the esthetician?

In studying the resources that are available in this discipline, I have found that what little material is available is broken down into various segments and does not give a complete picture of the benefits this great branch of medicine offers. There are few resources that explain how we can benefit from understanding the meridians that run up, down and across the face, or how Chinese herbal remedies and single herbs can help solve many skin concerns without using prescription drugs, harsh peels or plastic surgery. Chinese herbs help solve the imbalances internally so that the skin glows on the outside because it is healthy on the inside.

I wrote this book because I felt that there was something missing when I was doing facials. I was helping my clients with their particular skin issues; however, I didn't feel that I was solving the root cause of their problems.

I felt like I was putting a Band-aid on a symptom but I hadn't addressed where the problem originated inside the body. Chinese medicine helps bring your clients' skin back to its healthy state and helps their skin remain looking young because their bodies are working at optimal level from the inside out.

I enjoyed doing facials and making people feel good, but I wanted to bring them beauty from the inside out. I wanted their skin to radiate, so I needed to address the core issues with their skin. If they had acne, I wanted to address the hormonal issue; if they were experiencing dry skin and the beginning of fine lines and wrinkles, I wanted to heal their skin from the inside out. I tried recommending basic vitamins like A, C and E along with zinc and alpha lipolic acid with no dramatic change to the skin. I even followed many of the skin gurus out there who say that they have to maintain healthy skin. I do recommend vitamins, Omega oils, DMAE, alpha lipolic acid and probiotics for maintaining the health of the skin, but nutrients were not the complete answer. I wasn't able to find the "missing link" until I studied traditional Chinese medicine. Then I found the answers and remedies, and how to give my patients health, vitality, beauty and well-being without the use of drugs or unnecessary surgeries. I am so passionate about what I have learned that I want to share my knowledge with other estheticians and assist them in giving their clients beautiful skin from the inside out.

This book is written differently than most books on traditional Chinese medicine. This one is written for the esthetician, and shows how this healing art can help you and your clients feel and look their best.

As estheticians, we are not permitted to diagnose skin conditions, but we can use traditional Chinese medicine to study the eight meridians that flow across the face; we then can suggest a classic herbal remedy for a specific condition. In this book I also will discuss some foods that will benefit your clients' skin, along with a whole chapter on soups that addresses certain skin issues and incorporates the theory of the five elements. I will also introduce an ancient exercise technique that will benefit the qi of the body; this exercise will also benefit the skin. The last item will be an acupressure massage technique that your clients can do at home to help tone their skin and soften their fine lines and wrinkles.

I hope this book will spark your interest in this amazing healing art, and some of you will read more on this fascinating subject Furthermore, I hope some will become Doctors of Oriental Medicine and experience the power and awe of this incredible discipline that has been used so effectively for more than 5,000 years.

Chapter 1

History of Traditional Chinese Medicine

Traditional Chinese medicine (TCM) is a branch of science that teaches how the body works by looking at it in a holistic manner. Using TCM, we look for signs of deficiency or excess by analyzing different aspects of the body, including the face, the tongue and the meridians, the paths of energy that travel through the body. TCM uses treatments like acupuncture, Chinese herbs and dietary recommendations to bring the body back to harmony. In order to grasp the concepts of TCM, it is helpful to review its historical roots in classical Chinese medicine.

For more information on acupuncture, see chapter 13, "Acupuncture."

For more information on Chinese herbs, see chapter 8, "Chinese Herbal Medicine."

Classical Chinese medicine (CCM) started about 5,000 years ago with the shaman, or medicine man. The medicine man not only treated illness, he studied the plants and herbs that grew in the area and classified them into different categories according to their energetic properties, such as hot and cold.

The medicine men gained respect in their communities and started moving away from the spiritual aspect of healing as they concentrated more on the scientific aspects of how the body becomes diseased. They looked to nature and discovered the five elements: wood, fire, earth, metal and water. The medicine men believed that man was a miniature universe and had the five elements within him. Because the elements in nature transform into each other and can work against each other, the elements must be in balance, as imbalance can cause disease.

Early in the third century B.C., two silk scrolls discovered inside an excavated tomb described the meridians. Shortly after this discovery, the Warring States Period (approximately 476B.C. - 221B.C.) began. During this period, the medicine men were able to actively study how the body works because of the many men who were injured in war. While studying the injured, the medicine men confirmed the existence of these paths of energy (meridians) and discovered how to assist the body's healing by sticking thin needles into those paths of energy. The medicine men also found that if a patient had severe pain, inserting needles around the painful area decreased the amount of pain and encouraged the healing process by stimulating blood circulation in the injured area.

> For more information on meridians, see chapter 3, "Meridians."

Once the benefit of using needles was discovered, CCM started incorporating acupuncture and the study of herbs as a means of healing.

The results of these studies have been documented through the years. Many herbs were categorized into their different properties and put into classic books like *Shang Han Lun: On Cold Damage, Translation & Commentaries* by Zhonqiing Zhang. Another classic, *The Yellow Emperor's Classic of Internal Medicine* by Ilza Veith, wrote about the theory of yin and yang, the five elements and how to diagnose and prevent disease. *The Yellow Emperor's Classic of Internal Medicine* is still read by most acupuncturists today with awe and wonder at the knowledge gained so long ago.

As CCM became more widely known and its popularity grew, schools began opening where students could study the science. CCM remained a respected and honored profession until the English invaded China. During the Opium Wars in the mid 1800's, the Chinese began to think that Western medicine was superior to their own. In order to avoid being left behind by progress, the Nationalist government banned CCM from all hospitals. For 30 years, the practice of CCM was forbidden. Many were killed or fled for their lives during this time if caught practicing. Many CCM doctors practiced underground or fled to other countries to continue in their profession.

In the 1960's, Mao Zedong, founder of the People's Republic of China, decided that the government should not continue to outlaw the use of CCM. He commissioned the top 10 medical doctors in China to take a survey of CCM. They created a standardized format for its application, which is now known as traditional Chinese medicine (TCM).

Today, when you study traditional Chinese medicine in China, you also study Western medicine because both modalities are used in the hospitals. It is very interesting to see how Chinese hospitals have integrated the best of Western medicine—its techniques and tests—with the best of TCM—acupuncture, herbs and dietary recommendations. Through this combined approach, China has brought healing and health to many.

It will be an exciting day when every hospital and clinic incorporates the best of the West with the best of East to bring about optimal health for all people.

Chapter 2

QI

"Every birth is a condensation, every death a dispersal. Birth is not a gain, death not a loss...when condensed, Qi becomes a living being, when dispersed, it is the substratum of mutations."
—*Zhang Zai*

Traditional Chinese medicine teaches that there is a vital energy in the universe known as qi (chee) that permeates all living things, and filters through nature, our homes and our businesses. Qi can bring harmony to the body if it is flowing smoothly, or it can cause disharmony and sickness if it is blocked or stagnated. An example of this concept is Feng Shui, the study of how qi flows in our homes and businesses.

Everything that is breathing, moving and vibrating does so because of qi. Qi allows our bodies to function. It is the energy that warms us, keeps our immune systems strong and our vital organs functioning properly. It keeps our heart beating, our lungs strong and our digestive tract working efficiently. Without qi, we would be lifeless.

The qi in our body is created from the congenital qi we inherit from our parents. That congenital qi is enhanced by the foods we eat, the fluids we drink and the air we breathe. If we are eating healthy foods that are full of nutrients and drinking fluids that are beneficial to our bodies, we are taking in good qi that will keep our bodies functioning at its best. However, if we eat non-nutritious foods and drink a lot of soda or other drinks with empty calories, we are not taking in good qi. In the long run we will feel tired, stressed and worn out.

Some people are born with deficient congenital qi, which would require nourishment of the body with liquids and super foods (greens, algae and other foods that are packed with nutrients) to build up the body's strength. Many teenagers and twenty-somethings can eat junk food and stay up all night without many consequences because they are sustained by their healthy congenital qi. When they reach their forties, however, all that unhealthy living will catch up with them and their bodies will start breaking down because they haven't produced an abundance of good, healthy qi with their earlier diet and lifestyle.

> "In our twenties we have the body we inherited; in our forties we have the body we made; and in our fifties we have the body we deserve because of the way we lived in our earlier years."
>
> —Paraphrased from unknown source

Qi is an invisible energy, yet it is responsible for the energy that helps push blood and oxygen through our circulation system, bringing vital nutrients to every cell in our bodies. When our cells get enough oxygen and nutrients they are able to perform at an optimal level. Oxygen is inhaled; carbon dioxide and waste are pushed out of the cells and eliminated. If the circulation of blood and qi is sluggish or deficient, carbon dioxide and waste builds up in the cells. This causes more toxins to build up, which hurts the cells and the organs.

There are numerous ways to counter this build-up and bring healing to our bodies, including the use of acupuncture and herbs. We'll discuss these concepts, as well as others, in later chapters.

Chapter 3

Meridians

Acupuncture points are located along invisible lines on the body called meridians. There are 12 main meridians on the body, connected to the body's various organs. Qi travels along these meridians, bringing health and harmony to all the internal organs.

Meridians are like a network of rivers or channels that flow throughout the body. If they are blocked, there is disharmony. It is the acupuncturist's job to find and remove the blocks and restore the body's harmony.

For more information on qi, see chapter 2, "Qi". For more information on acupuncture, see chapter 11, "Acupuncture".

The 12 main meridians are as listed in **Table 3.1**.

Six of the 12 main meridians, and two additional meridians traverse the face:

- Gallbladder
- Stomach
- Small intestine
- Large Intestine
- Bladder
- Triple warmer
- Ren
- Du

We will discuss each of these in detail in the following sections.

Table 3.1

The table below gives a more systematic list of the meridans:

Meridian name/organ	Yin/Yang	Arm/Leg	5 elements
Lung	Major Yin	Arm	Metal
Pericardium	Yin	Arm	Fire
Heart	Minor Yin	Arm	Fire
Large Intestine	Yan	Arm	Metal
Triple Warmer	Minor Yang	Arm	Fire
Small Intestine	Major Yang	Arm	Fire
Kidney	Minor Yi	Leg	Water
Spleen	Major Yin	Leg	Earth
Liver	Yin	Leg	Wood
Stomach	Yang	Leg	Earth
Bladder	Major Yang	Leg	Water
Gallbladder	Minor Yang	Leg	Wood

Gallbladder Meridian

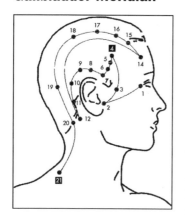

The gallbladder meridian begins beside the eye, travels around the ear and the side of the head, down the side of the body and leg to the end of the nail of the fourth toe.

The function of the gallbladder is to store and secrete bile into the digestive tract to aid digestion. Eating too many greasy, fatty foods can cause disharmony to this channel, which can result in eczema or breakouts. Emotionally, the gallbladder is related to the liver and is affected by constant anger, frustration, resentment and worry. These emotions can cause blockages in the channel resulting in migraines, nausea and digestive problems. Massaging the web of the fourth toe can help alleviate some of the pain, break up the stagnation and move the qi downward.

When looking at the face for disharmony in the gallbladder, look at the front of the ear or behind the ear for any breakouts, redness, scaly skin or eczema. You can also look at end of the eyebrow for any breakouts, congestions or redness. These signs are caused by an excess of heat in the gallbladder meridian. Herbs to help alleviate these symptoms are gardenia flower (Zhi Zi) and gentiana (Long Dan Cao).

The gallbladder is connected to the liver anatomically as well as with the meridians. Both organs manifest themselves around the eye area, so any heat, itching or redness around the eye shows excess heat in the liver/gallbladder organs. If wrinkles appear on the outer side of the eye it is a sign that there is disharmony in the liver. Herbs such as wolfberries (Gou Qi Zi) or white Chrysanthemum flower (Ju Hua) are beneficial in reducing this.

Stomach Meridian

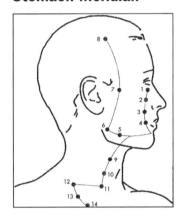

The stomach meridian begins under the pupil of the eye and descends down the front of the face to the edge of the mouth, up the cheek to the forehead and down the neck. From the jaw line it descends to the neck, crosses the chest, the abdomen, the front lateral side of the leg and ends at the second toe.

The function of the stomach is to receive food and break it down so it can be sent to the small intestine. The stomach meridian's function is to send the food downward for further processing.

If there is disharmony in this meridian, manifestations can include hiccups, nausea, vomiting and acid regurgitation. You may also see breakouts on the sides of the mouth and on the cheek. These breakouts are different from most papules because they are red and inflamed but do not contain much pus. If the client has a breakout along the mouth and the jaw line, this is a sign of heat and dampness in the stomach and large intestine. The large intestine meridian crosses the jaw line with the stomach so heat has to be removed from both the stomach and large intestine. Coptis (Huang Lian) is very good for clearing heat out of both these organs. Rhubarb (Da Huang) is also beneficial if the breakout is due to constipation and toxins in the large intestine because it drains all the heat and the dampness from the body through the large intestine.

The stomach and pancreas both manifest themselves around the mouth, so any lines around the mouth indicate disharmony in the stomach. Aloe Vera is excellent for nourishing the stomach as well as the whole digestive tract.

Small Intestine Meridian

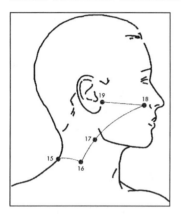

The small intestine meridian begins on the lateral side of the little finger, follows up the arm and crosses the back of the shoulder. It then goes on a zigzag course across the back of the shoulder to the side of the spine, and then to the cheek, where it finishes in front of the ear.

The function of the small intestine is to receive partially digested food from the stomach, extract the nutrients and send the impurities down to the large intestine or bladder for excretion. Too much raw food will cause dampness and whiteheads on the cheeks, while too many spicy or hot foods will cause pustules and inflammation.

Disharmony in the small intestine meridian appears as fine lines that start at the jaw bone about an inch lateral to the stomach meridian and run up the face toward the cheek. The length and deepness of the line depends on the severity of the deficiency.

Large Intestine Meridian

The large intestine meridian begins on the lateral side of the index finger, travels up the posterior lateral side of the arm and crosses the shoulder joint to ascend the lateral side of the neck, crossing the face to end on the side of the nose.

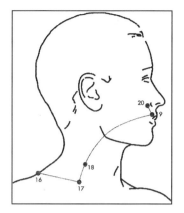

The function of the large intestine (or colon) is to receive waste from the small intestine, refine it to extract further nutrients and fluids and eliminate the rest. In dealing with excretion of waste, it is the most important meridian. If your clients are eating unhealthy foods, it will show up as blackheads and congestion on the side of the nose. The large intestine meridian also deals with negative thoughts like depression, anxiety and self-loathing. Therefore, skin breakouts can be caused by improper eating habits but also by negative emotions. Louise L. Hay, author of *You Can Heal Your Life*, says the cause of acne is "not accepting or disliking of self."

Signs of congestion in the large intestine may show at the sides of the nose, jaw line or forehead. This can be caused by recent antibiotic use, because an antibiotic will kill all the bacteria in your body, as well as the bacteria in your intestinal tract. This can be beneficial, but it can also cause problems when the bacteria begin to grow back, as it is usually the bad bacteria.

The large intestine is connected to the lungs; symptoms manifest on the nose, so dryness on the sides of the nose indicates dryness of the lungs or the large intestine. The lung meridian does not run on the face but it shows up on the medial area of the cheek

> The concept of Yin and Yang will be further explained in chapter 4, "Ying and Yang."

close to the nose. Rosacea usually shows up in that area because it is a sign of yin deficiency in the stomach or the lungs. If it is a lung yin deficiency, American ginseng is very good for nourishing the lungs and ophiopogon tuber (Mai Meng Dong) is very good for nourishing the yin of both the stomach and the lungs.

Bladder Meridian

The bladder meridian is the longest meridian of the body. It starts at the inner corner of the eye and crosses the scalp; descends the

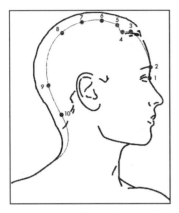

back, following the sides of the spinal column; follows the posterior center of the leg, down the lower half of the leg, where it moves to the outer side of the ankle and ends on the lateral side of the big toe.

The function of the bladder is to store urine and control excretion. It receives bodily fluids from the small intestine and large intestine and is influenced by the kidneys. When the eyes are puffy or have dark circles under them, it is usually an indication of eating a lot of salty food or drinking insufficient amounts of water. The swelling in the eye will usually show up in the upper inner eye. If there are dark circles under the eyes this indicates a yin deficiency in the kidneys, because the bladder and kidneys are connected. Two herbs that nourish the kidney and help with dark circles under the eyes include Lily Bulb (Bai He) and Mulberry mistletoe stems (Sang Ji Sheng).

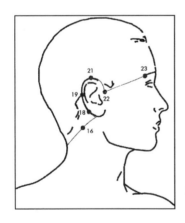

Triple Warmer Meridian

The triple warmer meridian starts on the nail of the ring finger; it then ascends the posterior side of the forearm and arm, passes over the shoulder and outer border of the neck, goes around the ear and ends at the outer corner of the eyebrow.

The triple warmer meridian is the first of three meridians that do not have a related organ. This meridian controls three areas of function.

Area	Responsible for:
Upper	Intake of breath above the diaphragm
Middle	Digestion
Lower	Excretion of waste

The triple warmer meridian is stimulated during lymphatic drainage. It helps get rid of toxins and waste from the lymph nodes. It is also very important in helping to bring nutrients and lymph fluid to the face. The gallbladder and the triple warmer meridians are connected so any problems around the ears can benefit from the same herbs such as gardenia (Zhi Zi), gentiana (Long Dan Cao) or hare's ear root (Chai Hu).

Ren Meridian

The ren meridian starts at the perineum and passes up the anterior midline of the body to the neck and upper jaw to the chin.

This meridian is the most yin of all the meridians and, along with the internal organs, is in charge of most female issues. Monthly facial breakouts are usually due to an imbalance in this meridian causing a hormonal breakout.

Most issues with the ren meridian manifest on the chin, which shows the health of the hormones in our body. If there is a breakout on the chin, there is too much heat being produced by the androgen hormone. There are two herbs that can help quench the fire: Chinese Dodder Seeds (Tu Si Zi) and Japanese Teasel Root (Xu Duan). A yin deficiency due to menopause usually shows up as lines on the chin, lines coming farther down on the nasal labial groove or a few lines on the jaw line below the sides of the mouth. Two herbs to help nourish the fine lines on the chin area are: Eclipta (Han Lian Cao) and Privet fruit (Nu Zhen Zi).

Du Meridian

The du meridian starts between the tip of the tailbone and anus; it then proceeds up the midline of the spinal column, passing over the head to end between the upper lip and gum.

This meridian is the most yang meridian because it is located on the back side of the body. This meridian is used to alleviate chronic back problems and to strengthen the mind and the body. We usually don't concentrate on this meridian for facial problems but we do look at it if the person has problems with the spine.

An esthetician's job is to be like a detective and find out the reason for the imbalances of the face. Most of our patients have more than one issue so it can be confusing until you break it down into a structured series of clues that will help you get to the core of the problem.

Meridians are your first clue. Once you know which meridian or meridians are affected, then you are going to figure out if there is too much heat, cold, dry or damp in that particular meridian and organ. This will help you figure out which herbs to use and what foods would benefit our clients.

Keep your Sherlock Holmes hat on as we begin with the second clue, ying and yang.

*All of the illustrations in this chapter were used with the permission of Sothys Paris, *www.sothys.com.*

Chapter 4

Yin and Yang

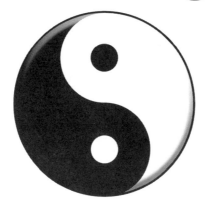

The basis of all concepts of traditional Chinese medicine lies in the concept of yin and yang. Yin and yang represent the opposite, or opposing manifestations, of everything in nature. The opposing concepts of yin and yang are viewed as interdependent and complementary. They create and control each other; one must be present for the other to exist. When there is an above, there has to be a below; if there is a front, there has to be a back. The constant interplay of yin and yang is the foundation of Chinese thinking. Everything in nature has been categorized according to yin and yang. For example:

Yin	Yang
Earth	Heaven
Female	Male
Night	Day
Interior	Exterior
Cold	Hot
Dark	Light
Quiet	Active
Lower Body	Upper Body (Face)

Yin and yang is represented by the black and white symbol which symbolizes the ancient Chinese understanding of how everything relates. The outer circle represents "everything." The black side of the circle represents yin and stands for "the dark side of the mountain." The white side of the circle represents yang and stands for "the bright side of the mountain".

The Body

The Chinese have adapted the yin and yang theory to the structure and function of the human body. In terms of anatomy, the body has been separated as follows:

Yin	Yang
Front	Back
Below the waist	Above the waist
Medial	Lateral

As for physiological functions, all the fluids of the body–such as blood, saliva, bodily fluids and hyaluronic acid–all pertain to yin while everything dealing with the functioning of the organs and the different systems pertain to yang.

Yin represents all the fluids of the body. It dries up as we get older and we begin to see dry, sensitive skin, fine lines and wrinkles. Red, blotchy skin and rosacea indicate that the cooling, moist properties of certain meridians are deficient, making the yang more exuberant and causing more heat in the skin. Hyperpigmentation (darkening of the skin) is a sign that the yin of the kidneys is weak and needs nourishment.

These manifestations appear because the systems involved are not working at optimal levels. The paleness occurs because the body is not manufacturing enough blood. Swollen skin is due to the lymph system not flowing well. Sagging skin indicates an overall deficiency in the body's yang and qi. The yang/qi is responsible for holding things in place; if the yang/qi is deficient you can experience prolapse of organs such as the uterus, intestines and rectum. Congested skin is a sign the body's metabolism is not working as well as it should.

The Face

To assess if there is a yin and yang deficiency, we can also look at the face.

Yin deficiency shows up on the face as:
1. Dry/ scaly skin
2. Wrinkles
3. Hyperpigmentation
4. Red, blotchy skin
5. Rosacea

Yang deficiency appears on the face as:
1. Pale skin
2. Swollen face or ankles
3. Sagging skin of the neck and eyelids
4. Clogged, congested pores

When analyzing the face, observe whether it is pale or red; swollen or gaunt; dry or oily; young or old. Look for signs that will tell you if your client's face is yin or yang. A pale and swollen face with dark circles under the eyes is a sign that the skin is yang deficient. In this case, use cinnamon or Ginseng herbal masks to invigorate the metabolism. If the face is hot, red and inflamed, it is either because the skin is yang exuberant due to an infection, or because the yin is too deficient to control the yang. If this is the case, cool it down with yin-type masks and similar products, including sulfur, kaolin clay and aloe.

In Chinese medicine, acne, or a red, inflamed breakout is a sign of heat, infection and dampness in the body. The redness is a sign of heat, while the pustules and papules are a sign of infection or dampness. Apply products such as tea tree oil, benzoyl peroxide or sulfur to kill the infection. All three of these products are antibacterial and will kill P acne bacteria spreading across the face.

The Metabolism

The skin metabolism is very important to the function of the skin. Sluggish metabolism of the skin results in congested, asphyxiated skin because the blood flow is slow and toxins build up in the cells, slowing down the metabolic process.

Yang-type products like cayenne pepper masks, pumpkin masks, cinnamon masks and glycolic acid invigorate the metabolism with heat. All of these products are hot and will help to break up cold and reduce excess water retention. However, these products shouldn't be used for too long because they can be very drying and can over-stimulate the face, causing it to become red, hot and overly sensitive. Once the circulation is working well and the complexion has a healthy glow, discontinue the invigorating masks. Then put on a balancing mask like a collagen fleece, gingko biloba mask or any other mask that is not too cold or too hot.

> It is very important to monitor the progress of your client. To avoid going over board and causing other problems, immediately change the regime once the skin condition has improved.

Meridians

The body's meridians have also been categorized as being either yin or yang. The yang meridians are the ones connected to the hollow organs of the body like the stomach and small and large intestines. The yin meridians are associated with the more solid organs like the liver, kidneys and heart.

The yang organs are hollow and in charge of processing food and eliminating waste, while the yin organs are more solid and responsible for transforming, storing and distributing food. The only yang organ that is not hollow is the gallbladder, which is considered to be both yin and yang. The yang meridians are your defense system against early illness, while the yin meridians are your defense from a chronic illness that has penetrated the interior of the body.

All the meridians that traverse the face are yang meridians, so they are responsible for carrying much of the qi and blood to and from the rest of the body. If the face is pale, it is usually a sign that the rest of the body is blood deficient. All the yang meridians either commence on the face and run down to the feet, or they begin on the hands and end on the face. All yin meridians either commence on the feet and run up to the chest, or they begin on the chest and run down the interior of the arm to finish on the hand. This is why many skin issues on the face occur with a sudden manifestation; red, hot and inflamed. By contrast, sores and other skin issues on the lower body have a slow manifestation; they tend to be chronic, swollen and more weepy or scaly in nature. The back is considered yang, while the front of the body is considered yin. The waist is the dividing line between upper body being more yang and the lower body being more yin. Consequently, if a skin condition shows up on the back and above the waist, it is more yang in nature; if it appears below the waist and on the front of the body, it is more yin.

Our first clue was found by looking at the meridians of the face to find out where the problem is inside the body. In this chapter, we have looked at yin and yang. For our next clue, we are going to look at the tongue.

Chapter 5

Tongue Diagnosis

One of the ways to diagnose the body and assess its imbalances is by looking at the tongue. There are six things to look at when assessing the tongue:

1. Color
2. Moisture
3. Coating
4. Fit in the Mouth
5. Appearance
6. Cracks

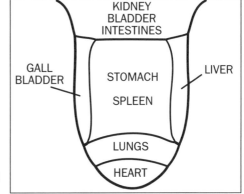

Color

The first detail to look at is color. Is it pale red, pale pink or red? If it is a pale red, it is healthy and it has enough qi and blood. If it is pale pink, the body is in a deficient state of qi and blood. If the tongue is red, it means there is excess heat in the body.

Moisture

The second detail to consider is moisture: whether it is dry, slightly moist or overly moist. If the tongue is dry, the fluids in the body are drying up because of too much heat. A slightly moist tongue is a healthy tongue. An overly moist tongue is a sign of excess dampness in the body and a sluggish lymph system.

Coating

The third detail to look at is the coating on the tongue:

- Is there a coating?
- Is it thick or thin?
- Is it white, yellow or red?

A thin white coating is normal, but a thick white coating means there is too much dampness in the body. Excess dampness is a sign of a sluggish metabolism or overuse of cold foods, which slow down the metabolism.

A yellow coating means there is dampness as well as heat in the body. Most of the time acne clients will have a red tongue with a thin or thick, yellow coating. The thicker the coating, the more dampness there is in the body. The deeper the yellow, the more heat there is than dampness.

A red tongue with no coating is a sign of yin deficiency. We see this tongue most often in clients who are menopausal, diabetic, taking very strong medications like antibiotics or smoking. When you see patients with this type of tongue, recommend they eat yin-rich foods (such as Aduki beans, cucumbers, soy beans, wood ear mushrooms, reiishi mushrooms and bitter melon) and avoid spicy, bitter or warming foods (such as ginger, curry, beef or alcohol).

Fit in the Mouth

The fourth detail to look at is how the tongue fits in the mouth; whether it is small or whether it is swollen and pushing on the sides of the mouth. If it is small and pale, it is a sign of blood deficiency. Foods that enrich the blood or a Chinese formula to build up the blood should be recommended. If the tongue is swollen, it is a sign that fluids are not draining well from the body; the lymph system is sluggish and there is too much dampness. Suggest warming foods to break up the dampness and stimulate the lymph system.

Appearance

The fifth detail we look at is how the tongue appears in different areas. The organs of the body are represented on the tongue as follows:

Area of Tongue	Represents
Tip	Heart
Behind Tip	Lungs
Middle	Spleen-pancreas, stomach
Sides	Liver and gallbladder
Back	Kidneys, bladder and large intestine

If you see redness only in a certain area, that lets you know where the heat is located. For example, a thick, yellow coating on the back of the tongue signifies there is heat and dampness in the lower part of the body.

Cracks

The sixth detail is cracks in the tongue. Are the cracks clustered in one area? Are they on one side, the middle, or is there one big crack all the way down the middle of the tongue?

Specific cracks on the tongue indicate that at some time the yin in that organ has been hurt or damaged.

Area of Tongue	Possible causes
Lung	Smoking (Pneumonia or Lung issues)
Stomach	Ulcer, Acid Reflux, Spicy Foods
Liver and Gallbladder	Anger, Stress, Alcohol, Spicy Foods, Cigarettes

Now let's review the three areas in which to look for clues:

1. The meridians: see which ones are affected and whether they are hot or cold. See chapter 3, "Meridians," for more information.

Food (such as a red life-saver) and drinks (such as coffee) can alter tongue color, so be mindful of this possibility when doing an assessment.

2. Yin and yang: see if the skin is too red and sensitive or too pale and swollen. See chapter 4, "Yin and Yang," for more information.

3. The tongue: see what it is telling us about the inside of the body.

Chapter 6

The Five Elements

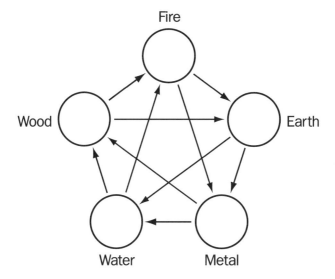

In addition to the meridian system and the theory of yin and yang, Chinese medicine has another way of categorizing life, nature and the human body. This system is called the five elements, which also presents all aspects of life in a balanced format. Everything in nature fits into five different categories or elements: wood, fire, earth, metal and water. **Table 6.1** shows the aspects involved in each of the five elements. "Five elements" is translated from the Chinese word "Wuxing." "Wu" stands for "five" and "xing" depicts something moving: a phase, transformation or change. The five elements have five dynamic qualities that interact with each other and balance each other out. For example, Feng Shui is the theory that peace and harmony can be created in a space if all five elements are present and in balance. A lot of estheticians use Feng Shui in their facial rooms by adding a plant

Table 6.1

Aspects of the Five Elements

Element	Aspect
Wood	Germination, wind, growth, harmony and flexibility, spring
Fire	Heat, Flaring upwards, fire, growth, summer
Earth	Growing, transformation, nourishing, dampness, and production, late summer
Metal	Strength, reaping, dryness, autumn
Water	Moisture, cold, descending, storing, winter

or tree (wood element), a fountain (water element), a mirror (metal element), a candle (fire element) and fresh flowers (earth element). The five elements can be applied not only to your home but your body, creating balance and harmony within yourself as well as with nature.

Each of the five elements of the body is associated with an internal yin and yang organ, sense, taste, color, season and emotion. The five elements are interconnected and each promotes the next; if one element is out of balance it will disrupt the other element. This imbalance will manifest itself in the individual through different signs and symptoms. It may show up in a certain facial color, sound in the voice, change in emotional state or disharmony in the functioning of connected organs. **Table 6.2** shows the categorization of phenomena according to the five elements.

For more information on Seasons, see chapter 7, "Colors and Seasons."

Now let's discuss aspects of each of the five elements in detail.

Wood

The wood element is associated with the liver and gallbladder. When liver function is stagnated, anger is common. When the liver is functioning properly, peace is felt. The color for the liver is green. If the face is tinged blue-green, it probably means there is stagnated blood, because the liver is in charge of the free flow of blood. The

Table 6.2

Five Element Phenomena Categorization

	Wood	Fire	Earth	Metal	Water
Flavors	sour	bitter	sweet	pungent	salty
Zang (yin organs)	liver	heart	spleen	lung	kidney
Fu (yang organs)	gall bladder	small intestine	stomach	large intestine	urinary
Senses	eye	tongue	mouth	nose	ear
Tissue	tendon	vessel	muscle	hair/skin	bone
Directions	east	south	center	west	north
Changes	germinate	grow	transform	reap	store
Color	green	red	yellow	white	black
Emotion	anger, depression, frustration	mania	worry, anxiety	grief	fear

blue-green color often shows up around the eye area, as the wood element manifests around the eyes. To break up stagnation of blood and improve circulation, eat red peppers, tomatoes and beets. To benefit the liver, drink a tea made with beet greens, dandelion and lemon.

The liver is the organ in charge of helping the body break down toxins. If the liver is sluggish or full of toxins like aspirin, medication, alcohol, cigarettes and processed food, it too will try to rid the body of toxins via the skin. When severe acne or chronic congestion occurs, there is usually a problem with elimination through the colon. To combat this, the liver should be detoxified so that toxins can be eliminated and the colon, lung, and liver can work in harmony. Chlorophyll is an excellent drink for detoxifying the liver. Naturopaths say that chlorophyll is very close to our blood content, so by drinking it we are bringing fresh oxygen to the organs and ridding our bodies of toxins. Chlorophyll by nature is very cold so people who always suffer from cold hands and feet should not take it because it will make them colder.

A few herbs that are also beneficial to the liver include white peony (Bai Shao Yao), radix bupleuri (Chai Hu), and mint (Bo He). A classic formula recommended for people under a lot of stress is called "free and easy wanderer" (Xiao Yao Wan).

Fire

The fire element rules the heart and small intestine. In Chinese medicine, the heart represents not only the actual heart organ, but one's emotional state. The Chinese believe that the heart not only circulates the blood, but also controls consciousness, spirit, sleep and memory. When our hearts are healthy, we are able to solve problems effortlessly and arrive at brilliant solutions. When our hearts are imbalanced, we feel confused and scattered, with either an excess of laughter or no laughter.

The emotion for the heart is joy, the sound is laughter and the color is red. When there is too much redness in the face, we need to think about the heart and recommend foods that are bitter; they have a descending and cooling quality and are cleansing to the heart and associated arteries.

The sense organ for the heart is the tongue. Some signs that the heart is imbalanced include stuttering, excessive talking and confused speech. Another sign is sores on the tongue. Some foods that are calming to the heart include mushrooms, brown rice, oats, jujube and a Chinese herb called Suan Zao Ren. Herbs such as chamomile, catnip, skullcap, passion flower and valerian are calming and very helpful when your mind is racing and you cannot go to sleep.

Earth

The earth element rules the stomach and the spleen-pancreas. The spleen and pancreas are both primarily responsible for digestion and distribution of food and nutrients. The qi energy created by the extracted nutrients from the food helps keep the body warm, healthy and fighting infection. The spleen-pancreas is also responsible for the formation of tissues.

When these organs are healthy, people are usually hard-working, practical and responsible. They like to nurture themselves and others.

They are strong, active and stable. They have good digestion and a hearty appetite. They are orderly and often excel at some artistic activity. When the spleen-pancreas is imbalanced the signs can include:

- Mental and physical exhaustion
- Depression
- Poor digestion
- Nausea
- Bloating
- Gas
- Distention
- Becoming tired after eating
- Poor appetite
- Loose stools
- Weight gain

The Earth element manifests itself around the mouth, and its color is yellow. If the client has fine lines around the mouth and has never smoked, there is probably an imbalance in the spleen-pancreas. If the client has a sallow complexion, it can be a sign of poor digestion.

The spleen-pancreas is affected by the emotion of worry. Worry causes our digestion to slow down and slows the release of enzymes from the pancreas.

The spleen-pancreas is considered the center of all the energy, so when the digestive system is not working, it affects the periphery of the body; usually the arms and legs. Therefore, another sign that the spleen-pancreas is not functioning properly is weak muscle tone and an underdevelopment of the muscles in children. The spleen-pancreas is also responsible for holding the internal organs in place, so prolapsed uteri, hemorrhoids, kidneys, stomach and intestines are all signs of a weak spleen-pancreas. This shows up on the face as sagging eyelids and jowls, and loose skin under the chin.

The Chinese have a wonderful herbal formula to tonify the spleen-pancreas. It is called "Si Jun Zi Tang," which literally translates into "the four gentlemen" because it consists of four different herbs. They are Panax ginseng, white atractylodes, poria and licorice. This herbal formula is great for anyone who has weak digestion and is even safe enough for children over the age of two.

Spices that help to tonify the spleen-pancreas are usually warming in nature; examples include ginger, cinnamon, cardamom, fennel and nutmeg. Some foods that can be added to the diet are carrots, sweet potatoes, parsnips, turnips, pumpkin, rutabagas, onions, leeks and barley. These foods should be cooked and, if possible, made into a soup or congee (Chinese porridge) so that they are easily digested and the nutrients are quickly absorbed in the small intestines.

Foods that should be avoided include raw vegetables and fruits, sweets and cooling foods such as tofu, spinach, tomato, blue-green algae, seaweed, all dairy products, refined sugars, processed foods and large rich meals. When we eat these foods while the spleen-pancreas is in a weakened state, it creates a moist sticky substance in the body that we call dampness. The dampness is the extra weight in the waist area, a heavy feeling in the body, congested skin, bloated stomach, mucus discharge from the nose and a foggy mind. It usually permeates every part of the body, making one feel sluggish, tired, bloated and depressed; other symptoms include a runny nose or a persistent phlegm cough, which is usually worse in the morning.

Metal

The metal element rules the lungs and large intestines. The lungs are responsible for breathing and the sense of smell. In Chinese medicine, we say that the lungs breathe in heavenly qi, which is mixed with the food qi and then becomes the acquired qi that travels all over the body. The lungs are considered to be the canopy that covers all the other internal organs; they are also the only internal yin organ that has direct contact with the outside world. It is the first organ that gets attacked by external pathogens. We usually know if we are catching a cold because we start to cough or get a stuffy nose. We say that the lung qi is responsible for producing the "Wei Qi," which is our "defensive qi" that protects us from external pathogens.

There are a couple of Chinese herbs that are used for those who often catch colds and suffer from weak immune systems; one is astralagus (Huang Qi), and the other is a famous herbal remedy called

"Yu Ping Feng San," which translates into "jade wind screen." Both are excellent if you are constantly sick or perspiring for no apparent reason.

The lung is also in control of the skin and the pores. The lung and large intestine meridians are targeted for treatment with any skin conditions because of their yin and yang connection. Dry skin is usually caused by an improper diet, excessive exercise, a hostile climate or a malfunctioning lung or large intestine. The other signs of dryness include itchy skin and dryness of the nose, lips, skin and throat. Some foods that are very nourishing to the dry skin are soy, spinach, barley, pear, apple, persimmon, sesame seed and almond. Those with dryness should use bitter, warming foods with caution because of their dispersing and warming actions; they can cause more dryness.

The emotions that affect the lungs are grief and sadness. When the lung qi is weak, there are usually problems "letting go" of an item or a relationship. Being disorderly, and losing possessions easily or holding onto them with unreasonable attachment are other issues that may arise. Repressed grief causes long-term contraction of the lungs, leading to problems with dispersing acquired qi and a build up of matter that causes congestion. In his book, *Healing With Whole Foods: Asian Traditions and Modern Nutrition*, Paul Pitchard states, that "virtually everyone with lung and colon problems, regardless of the source of the problem, has unresolved sadness that needs to be addressed." Sharing such feelings with others can help dissipate them. Also, the expansive nature of pungent foods can help to clear out mucus from the lungs.

The lungs and colon are also affected by a poor diet, smoking, consuming too much meat and dairy products and eating too little fiber. These actions can cause toxins to build up in the colon, and when they can not be eliminated through the colon, they are sent to another excretory organ: the skin. The body has three ways to rid itself of toxins:

1. Excrete feces via the colon
2. Expel urine via the bladder
3. Sweat via pores in the skin

Water

The water element rules the kidneys and the bladder. These two organs are responsible for the body's water metabolism. The Chinese believe the kidneys are also responsible for sexual development, bones and the qi we inherit from our parents ("Jing"). The kidneys are seen as the root and foundation of the body; they rule the lower part of the body, provide warmth and energy and are the foundation of all the body's yin and yang qualities. The Chinese call the kidneys the "palace of fire and water" because of their yin and yang connection. The kidney yin affects the whole body's yin, which includes all the moisturizing fluids. The kidney yang affects the entire body's yang, which includes all its functions and energy. When a person has healthy kidneys, they are active yet calm; courageous but gentle; and accomplish a great deal without stress. They also balance assertiveness with the capacity for nurturing.

The kidneys open up to the ears, so any problems with hearing or ringing in the ear are considered to be signs of a kidney disharmony.

The emotion that is associated with the kidneys is fear or terror, which is why when one is in absolute fear they will unconsciously urinate on themselves. If somebody is always jumpy or constantly talking about being scared, the kidneys and adrenals are becoming deficient. Some general symptoms of a kidney imbalance include:

- Bone problems, especially those of the knees, back and teeth
- Hearing loss and ear infections
- Head and hair problems, including hair loss, split ends and premature graying
- Urinary, sexual or reproductive problems
- Poor growth and development of the mind and body
- Premature aging
- Excessive fear and insecurity

The kidneys usually manifest imbalances from a state of deficiency in yin, yang or qi. Refer to **Tables 6.3**, **6.4** and **6.5** for a listing of the signs and the nourishing foods and herbs related to them.

Table 6.3
Yin Deficiency in the Kidneys

Signs	Ringing in the ear, dry skin, dry throat, night sweats, weak legs, malar flush on the face.
Nourishing Foods	Tofu, millet, barley, soy, black beans, mung beans, watermelon and other melons, blackberries, mulberries, blueberries, water chestnuts, wheat germ, seaweeds, spirulina, black sesame seeds, sardines, eggs, aloe and cheese.
Nourishing Herbs	Marshmallow root, rehmannia root (Shu Di Huang), fleeceflower root (He Shou Wu), and black mushrooms (esp. "Black Fungus" or "Wood Ear")

Table 6.4
Yang Deficiency in the Kidneys

Signs	Cold hands and feet, cold shoulders, pale complexion, dark circles under the eyes, weak knees and lower back, mental fatigue, lack of sexual desire, frequent urination, edema and lack of will power and direction.
Nourishing Foods	Cloves, ginger, cinnamon bark, fennel seeds, black peppercorns, walnuts, black beans, everything in the onion family (garlic, onions, chives, leeks), chicken, lamb, trout and salmon

Table 6.5
Qi Deficiency in the Kidneys

Signs	Lower back weakness, weak knees, frequent urination and lethargy
Nourishing Foods	Oyster shell calcium, Chinese yams (Shan Yao)
Nourishing Herbs	Astralagus (Huang Qi) Licorice (Gan Cao) Ginseng

Each of the five elements is associated with a certain color and season. We will explore this is the next chapter.

Chapter 7

Colors and Seasons

Colors

Each of the five elements we discussed in the previous chapter are associated with a particular color. The colors are categorized as follows:

Element	Wood	Fire	Earth	Metal	Water
Color	green	red	yellow	white	black

The wood element is associated with the color green, so all your green foods benefit the liver and gallbladder. These include spinach, broccoli, dandelion greens, kale, bok choy, brussels sprouts, green beans, collard greens, mustard greens, bitter melon and green peppers.

The fire element is associated with the color red, so all foods that are red in color, including tomatoes, red peppers, beets, strawberries and cranberries benefit the heart and small intestine. Western doctors are now saying that lycopene—which is derived from tomatoes—is very beneficial for the heart because of all its antioxidants. The Chinese have known this for centuries.

The earth element is associated with the colors yellow and orange, so foods like pumpkin, squash, butternut squash, yellow peppers, peaches, nectarines, papaya, pineapple, mangoes and corn benefit the spleen-pancreas and stomach.

The metal element is associated with the color white, so foods like cauliflower, pears, apples, white asparagus, bamboo shoots, lotus root, white onions, white turnip and garlic benefit the lungs and large intestine.

The water element is associated with the color blue-black, so foods like plums, blackberries, blueberries, black beans, eggplant, black kale, black sesame seeds, seaweeds, black fungus and any black mushrooms benefit the kidneys and bladder.

The more colors we add to our meals, the greater the harmony will be among all the elements within our bodies.

Seasons

Each season of the year is associated with a certain element. It is during that season the associated organ is most vulnerable, so we should eat more foods in that color to nourish that organ and keep it healthy. Also, if we eat according to the seasons, it will be the time when most of the foods for that organ are in season.

The wood element is associated with spring. This is the period when most people break out in rashes or have eczema flare-ups. This is a good time to do a liver detoxification and to eat simple dishes with lots of green vegetables.

The fire element is associated with summer. This is when people get overheated and have problems with their blood pressure. During this time, it is best to eat foods like roasted red peppers, watermelon or chilled tomato soups to bring back the fluids lost during perspiration. Make sure clients drink plenty of water and wear sunscreen.

The earth element coincides with the end of summer and the beginning of fall when all the gourds are in season and peaches and nectarines are shipped from Georgia. Be careful not to eat too much sweet, rich food during this time. A nice juicy peach is great, but don't overindulge. Digestion will be weak, and if you suffer from digestion issues this will be the time when they flare up. Make a soup of pumpkin and ginger if you are feeling fatigued and worn out. The spleen-pancreas likes light soups during this time because they are already broken down and not hard on the digestion.

The metal element is associated with the fall, when the weather starts to change and the air becomes crisp. The lungs are affected by the dryness in the air and people are prone to colds and flu. Make sure to keep your chest and throat covered during this time if your lungs are your weakness. To nourish your lungs, eat plenty of foods that are white; like pears, cauliflower, onions and garlic. Garlic is also a great antibacterial, anti-fungal and antiviral, so it will also boost your immune system. An elephant garlic bulb roasted and spread on fresh baked whole wheat bread is great for the whole family, and a bowl of French onion soup without the cheese will make your lungs very happy during the fall weather.

The water element is associated with winter, a time to eat warm soups with everything thrown in, including lamb, beef and all the root vegetables like parsnips, turnips, rutabagas, leeks and beans. Because the kidneys are the root of both yin and yang in the body, make sure the food is warm in seasoning as well as in temperature. Since this is the time when all the aches and pains start flaring up, be sure to keep the lower back warm. Cod liver oil and the omega oils are beneficial for the kidneys and for body aches. It is also beneficial to eat figs, plums, and a lot of nuts like walnuts, chestnuts, pecans and almonds during this time.

See **Table 7.1** for facial conditions seem more frequently during particular seasons.

Table 7.1
Skin Problems Associated with Each Season

Spring	Summer	Fall	Winter
Rashes	Flushed face	Dryness	Dryness
Acne	Rosecea	Scaliness	Dark circles
Allergic Reactions	Eczema		Hyperpigmentation
	Psoriasis		Hormonal breakouts
			Edema

The right foods are very beneficial, but they are not always strong enough to solve the core issue. Chinese herbs help nourish the body at the core and bring the body back to balance. In the next chapter, we will delve into the wonderful world of Chinese herbs. This subject is so extensive it will take an eternity to master it. The next chapter is just a glimpse or a taste of this vast subject. Hopefully it will peak your interest to study more and see how we can help our clients with herbs instead of harsh prescriptions.

Chapter 8

Chinese Herbal Medicine

Chinese herbal medicine is another tool that acupuncturists use to heal their patients. Acupuncture helps release blockages in the meridians, while herbal medicine treats the main cause of the internal imbalances. Using acupuncture and herbs gives the patient a more comprehensive treatment. Most of the classic formulas that are prescribed today date back to around 200 B.C. when a famous herbalist named Zhang Zhong Jing wrote *Shang Han Lun*, the first book to focus on prescriptions of individual herbs, which is still used to this day.

Herbal formulas are made up of roots, barks, twigs, stems, leaves, seeds and flowers of many plants both wild and cultivated. Some formulas also use minerals and animal products. Herbal medicines are usually taken as a "recipe" or prescription, consisting of a combination of herbs to solve any imbalances in the body. These prescriptions are based on the Chinese diagnoses of disease, while Western herbs are usually prescribed as single herbs using Western diagnosis.

Herbs can be prepared in a variety of different ways. They can be taken as pills, tinctures or decoctions. The pill form seems to be the easiest for most Americans, but the herbs can also be ingested in dried form in tea or capsules. To make the pill form, the herb is freeze-dried and pulverized into a powder, then placed into capsules that can be swallowed. The tincture preparation is a concentrated liquid extract of herbs in alcohol. This preparation is very easy to take but should be avoided by people who have excess heat in their bodies or an addiction to alcohol.

Herbs are categorized based on their main action, such as regulating qi, tonifying qi, tonifying blood, draining dampness, clearing heat, clearing blood heat, tonifying yang, tonifying yin, extinguishing wind, calming the spirit and removing food stagnation. There are many different categories of actions for herbs, but as an esthetician you really only need to concentrate on nine of them:

- Heat-Clearing
- Damp-Draining
- Heat-Clearing and Damp-Draining
- Qi-Tonifying
- Yin-Tonifying
- Yang-Tonifying
- Blood-Tonifying
- Blood-Invigorating
- Herbs that Stop Bleeding

Herbs from these categories help different conditions of the face and body. Most of the formulas are a mixture of herbs from the various categories.

> Keep in mind that some clients will have a combination of different symptoms at the same time.

1. **Heat-Clearing** herbs clear heat—such as dry throat, red face, and red eyes—from the body. They are cold in nature and are anti-pyretic, anti-inflammatory and antimicrobial. They are used when the client has a fever, slight sweating and redness all over the face. Examples of this type of herb are gardenia (Zhi Zi) and cassia seeds (Jue Ming Zi).

2. **Damp-Draining** herbs are used when your client has several papules, blackheads and congestion on the face but there is not any inflammation, redness or heat. Most of these herbs are acrid, warm and aromatic. They are used to dry up the excessive dampness in the body showing up on the client's face. One of the main reasons for the congestion on the face is a slow metabolism. The client may be eating an excessive amount of dairy products and raw foods. A few

examples of damp-draining herbs include cardamon (Bai Dou Kou), black atractylodes (Cang Zhu) and poria (Fu Ling).

3. **Heat-Clearing and Damp-Draining** herbs clear excess heat and relieve toxicity in the body. These herbs are usually bitter and cold. They are anti-pyretic, anti-microbial and anti-inflammatory. They are used frequently on acne patients that have red, congested, and inflamed skin. An example of these types of herbs is skullcap (Huang Qin), sophora root (Ku Shen) and rhizome.

Tonifying herbs are those that strengthen or supplement an area of the body that is deficient or weakened. They also strengthen the body's defenses against disease. Tonics are used in treating patterns of deficiency in qi, yin, yang and blood. Most of the time, when the body is qi deficient, it is also yang deficient, and when it is yin deficient, it is also blood deficient.

4. **Qi-Tonifying** herbs are usually sweet and warming in nature. They are used for clients who have pale, tired, stressed skin. In this case, the skin may not be exfoliating fast enough and the metabolism of the skin may be slow. Wonderful examples of qi tonifying herbs include Korean ginseng (Ren Shen) , Chinese yams (Shan Yao), and astralagus (Huang Qi)

5. **Yin-Tonifying** herbs tonify the fluids of the body. As we get older, our fluids start to dry up; for example, this happens to the glycominoglycans in the dermis of the skin which give skin that plump, healthy look. When the yin of the body starts to be depleted, the skin starts to look gaunt and begins to wrinkle. Tonifying yin helps build up the glycoaminoglycans and alleviate skin dryness. Yin tonifying herbs regulate fluid metabolism and are sweet and cold in nature. A few examples of yin tonics include American ginseng (Xi Yang Shen) and the lily bulb (Bai He).

6. **Yang-Tonifying** herbs tonify the yang of the body. The yang herbs are very much like the qi tonifying herbs; they are warming in nature. A few benefits include:
   - Warming of the kidney yang which helps to rev up the libido in both men and women

- Increase in fertility (they are used in formulas for infertility)

A few examples of yang tonics include:

- Velvet of a young deer antler (Lu Rong). It is very expensive, but is very effective in treating exhaustion or a chronic condition that is depleting the body. This herb can be taken by itself. Put a few shavings in about 32 oz of hot water, let it steep and drink it during the day. The taste is very pleasant.
- Morinda root (Ba Ji Tian). It is highly nutritious and is used in tonic formulas for strengthening the body. It is often used to increase sexual strength in men and women, particularly for impotence and infertility.

7. **Blood-Tonifying** herbs are used when clients are blood-deficient. If they are not getting enough blood to the facial tissues, they are also not getting enough oxygen, which causes the face, lip and nails to look pale. The skin is not functioning at optimal level; everything slows down because all the vital nutrients the skin needs to function, heal and repair itself are lacking. This is the first sign of aging. To help clients combat the signs of aging we need to give them herbs that tonify their blood and qi, so the skin can start working at an optimal level again. Most of these herbs strengthen the body to improve its nutrition, thereby indirectly increasing the number of circulating blood cells. Several of these herbs are rich in nature and can be hard on the digestion if taken alone, so they are usually mixed with other herbs. Examples of blood-enhancing herbs include Chinese angelica (Dang Gui), white peony (Bai Shao Yao), jujubes (Da Zao) and wolfberries (Gou Qi Zi).

8. **Blood-Invigorating** herbs are used primarily to assist the flow of blood that has been retarded, blocked or made static. They are used when the skin has experienced trauma or surgery. A bruise is an accumulation of blood that is stagnant; blood-invigorating herbs help break up bruising and help the skin heal at a quicker rate. They help break up dead blood vessels and invigorate new blood to the area, which also brings oxygen and nutrients to help the skin heal. These herbs are usually acrid in nature. A few examples include

salvia root (Dan Shen), frankincense (Ru Xiang), red peony (Chi Shao) and safflower flower (Hong Hua).

9. **Herbs that Stop Bleeding** are used to treat trauma. These herbs should not be used alone but in conjunction with others, such as blood-invigorating herbs. They are usually bitter in nature. Examples of herbs that are used extensively after trauma include notoginseng root (Sang Qi) and cattail pollen (Pu Huang). Both of these herbs stop bleeding and also move the blood. They are both very effective in speeding up recovery after surgery or after experiencing any form of traumatic injury.

If you are interested in learning more on the subject of Chinese herbs, there are several books on the subject, including *Between Heaven and Earth* by Harriet Beinfield and Efrem Korn; and *The Web That Has No Weaver* by Ted J. Kaptchuk.

Chinese herbs are very potent. I recommend visiting an acupuncture physician who can mix a formula that will address your particular needs. The process of writing an herbal prescription is both a science and an art. It has to address the patient's concerns, but all the herbs also have to work together harmoniously so the body will heal. When I first tried to write up formulas for my patients, my teachers told me that I was not allowing the herbs to work together to bring my patients back to health. I have improved, however, but I know I will spend the rest of my life becoming skilled at making formulas for my patients.

In the next chapter, I will show you pictures of common herbs so that you can recognize them when you are shopping.

Chapter 9

Chinese Herbs

This chapter includes a list of common herbs that are extremely beneficial. The most common applications and possible results are listed.

> The herbs and foods mentioned in this chapter are included in the soups we will be discussing in chapter 15, "Soups for the Skin."

Aduki Beans (Chi Xiao Dou)

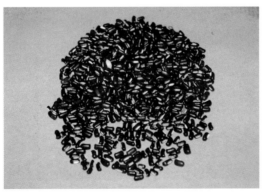

Applications and results:
1. Removes dark circles under the eyes
2. Treats acne
3. Treats edema
4. Moves blood

Angelica Root (Dang Gui)

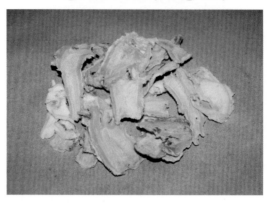

Applications and results:
1. Tonifies the blood to treat pale skin
2. Addresses irregular menses
3. Regenerates the skin
4. Alleviates acne and congested skin

Anise Stars (Ba Chio)

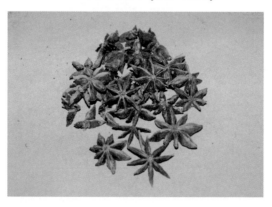

Applications and results:
1. Alleviates cough
2. Helps with digestion
3. Tonifies the spleen-pancreas
4. Treats sallow skin

Astralagus (Huang Qi)

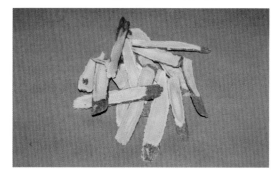

Applications and results:
1. Addresses spleen-pancreas deficiency
2. Treats sagging skin
3. Strengthens weak immune system
4. Tonifies qi and blood
5. Reduces edema
6. Promotes the discharge of pus from skin

Bitter Melon (Ku Gua)

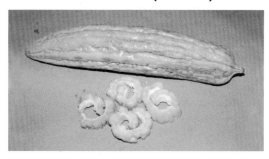

Applications and results:
1. Lowers blood sugar (for diabetics)
2. Treats psoriasis
3. Treats acne
4. Relieves common cold
5. Treats rosacea
6. Treats couperose (dilation of red blood vessels)
7. Gets the digestive juices flowing

Black Fungus (Bai Mu Er)

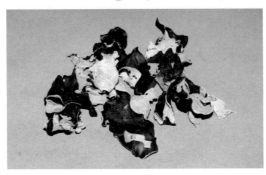

Applications and results:
1. Tonifies yin
2. Tonifies the kidneys
3. Addresses dark circles under the eyes
4. Alleviates hyperpigmentation
5. Removes fine lines around the eyes
6. Treats dry skin
7. Strengthens weak knees and lower back

Black Sesame Seeds (Hei Zhi Ma)

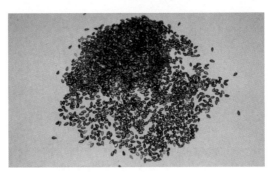

Applications and results:
1. Nourishes and tonifies the liver and kidneys
2. Removes fine lines around the eyes
3. Removes dark circles under the eyes
4. Treats dry skin
5. Addresses gray hair

Burdock Root (Niu Bong)

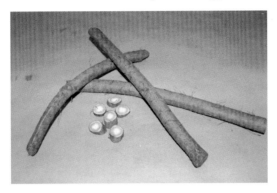

Applications and results:
1. Detoxifies the body
2. Treats acne
3. Treats breakouts

Cardamon Seeds (Bai Dou Kou)

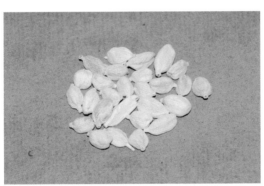

Applications and results:
1. Alleviates skin congestion
2. Promotes the movement of qi
3. Eliminates stagnation
4. Warms the middle to help with digestion

Chrysanthemum Flower (Ju Hua)

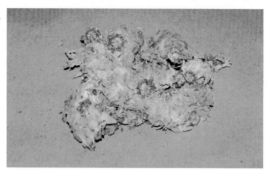

Applications and results:
1. Treats red eyes
2. Treats itchy eyes
3. Removes fine lines around the eyes
4. Alleviates headache

Hosuwu (He Shou Wu)

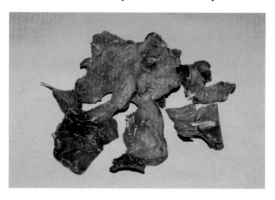

Applications and results:
1. Tonifies liver and kidney
2. Treats fine lines around the eye area
3. Eliminates dark circles
4. Addresses gray hair
5. Alleviates wind rash
6. Treats pale skin

Jujubes, or Chinese Dates (Da Zao)

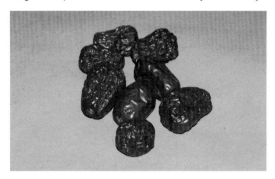

Applications and results:
1. Tonifies the spleen and qi
2. Helps with fatigue
3. Nourishes the blood
4. Calms the spirit, reduces irritability

Korean Ginseng (Ren Shen)

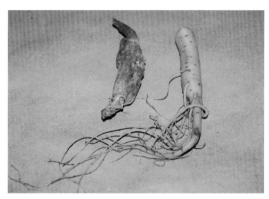

Applications and results:
1. Strengthens the spleen-pancreas
2. Generates fluids to treat dry skin
3. Improves qi and addresses blood deficiency
4. Treats sagging of the skin
5. Benefits the heart and calms the spirit

Licorice Cooked in Wine (Zhi Gan Cao)

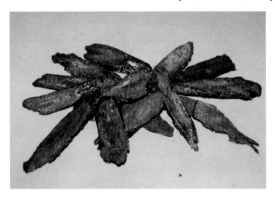

Applications and results:
1. Tonifies the spleen-pancreas
2. Moistens the lungs and stops cough
3. Serves as an adrenal tonic
4. Alleviates dry skin

Lily Bulb (Bai He)

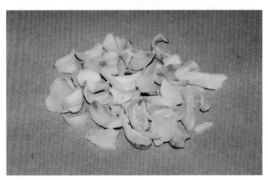

Applications and results:
1. Addresses dry skin
2. Treats rosacea
3. Alleviates insomnia
4. Treats dry throat and cough
5. Calms the spirit

Lotus Root (Ou Jie)

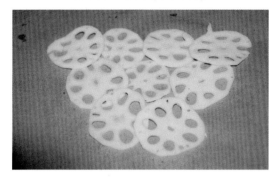

Applications and results:

1. Breaks up bruises after surgery
2. Helps with traumatic injury
3. Clears heat
4. Treats red face
5. Beautifies the skin

Mung Beans (Lu Dou)

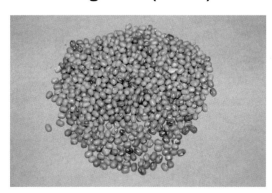

Applications and results:

1. Clears summer heat
2. Treats edema
3. Treats hyperpigmentation
4. Addresses oily skin

Poria (Fu Ling)

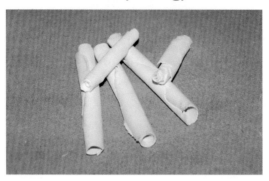

Applications and results:
1. Treats edema
2. Alleviates skin congestion
3. Strengthens the spleen-pancreas
4. Calms the spirit
5. Promotes weight loss

Salvia Root (Dan Shen)

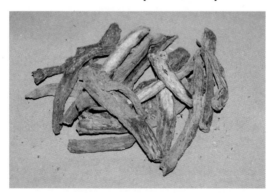

Applications and results:
1. Moves blood and breaks up stagnation
2. Clears heat
3. Stops irritability
4. Treats irregular menses
5. Alleviates insomnia

Shitake Mushrooms (Xiang Gu)

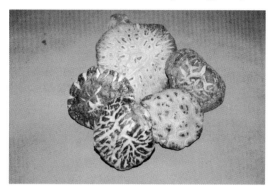

Applications and results:
1. Nourishes the kidneys
2. Addresses dry skin
3. Serves an anti-aging function
4. Treats wrinkles
5. Treats tumors
6. Addresses qi deficiency
7. Alleviates fatigue
8. Improves blood circulation

White Radish (Bai Lou Be)

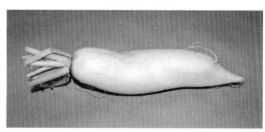

Applications and results:
1. Detoxifies the body
2. Treats hyperpigmentation
3. Treats acne
4. Treats edema

Wintermelon (Dong Gua)

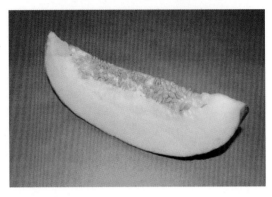

Applications and results:
1. Clears heat and expels pus
2. Treats acne
3. Alleviates red skin
4. Promotes weight loss
5. Treats urinary tract infections

Wolfberries (Gou Qi Zi)

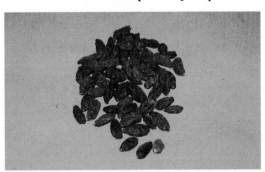

Applications and results:
1. Nourishes and tonifies the liver and kidneys
2. Improves yin and treats blood deficiency
3. Brightens the eyes
4. Treats fine lines around the eye area
5. Addresses pale skin

Chapter 10

Tastes

Traditional Chinese medicine applies the healing properties of food to correct disharmonies in the body. After carefully studying imbalances in the body, specific foods can be chosen to bring about healing. The Chinese believe that the qi of the body can be improved with the foods you eat and the teas you drink.

Chinese nutrition differs from Western nutrition in that it does not deal with the biochemical nature of food but rather its energetic qualities; such was warming, cooling, drying and lubricating. Food is also broken down by taste, because certain tastes stimulate different organs. For example:

- Sour foods stimulate the liver/gallbladder.
- Sweet foods stimulate the pancreas/stomach.
- Salty foods stimulate the kidney/bladder.
- Bitter foods stimulate the heart/small intestine.
- Pungent foods stimulate the lung/large intestine.

Each of the tastes also have different effects on the body, all of which should be incorporated into your diet to bring about harmony. The Western idea of a balanced meal is different than the Chinese idea. The Chinese look at the energetic qualities of the food and how they affect the harmony of our bodies, and try to have each taste present at every meal.

Sour

The sour taste has an absorbing, astringent function. It stops abnormal discharges of fluid from the body, like excessive sebum on the face. Examples of sour foods are vinegar and lemons. Anybody who has papules and congestion on the face should drink a hot cup of water with one-half of a lemon first thing in the morning. The hot water and lemon stimulate the liver to release bile, which breaks up fats.

Clients who are overweight from overeating and have voracious appetites should eat the pungent cooling foods instead of the warming ones, because those foods will curtail hunger. If the client is overweight and hardly eats, suggest warming foods to rev up the metabolism and help the body burn calories.

Sweet

The sweet taste has the function of tonifying, harmonizing and calming. In cases of fatigue and deficiency of qi, blood, yin or yang, sweet substances have a strengthening action. This is why we crave sweets when we are feeling low or tired. When sweet foods build up the yin of the body, fluids build up that can benefit a client who has very dry skin. The problem is some people have the tendency to eat too much sugar, and instead of strengthening the body, it causes damage. Examples of sweet foods are yams, carrots, turnips and winter squash. If you have a sluggish metabolism and feel tired most of the day, rather than eating a candy bar, add some of these natural foods to stimulate your pancreas to release its enzymes.

Salty

The salty taste has the function of softening and dissolving hardness. It also moistens and lubricates the intestines. Lumps, masses and cysts can be dissolved with salty substances like seaweed. Also, in cases of constipation, one can drink a cup of warm salt water to lubricate the intestines and promote evacuation.

Bitter

The bitter taste has the function of drying dampness and phlegm. The dispersing properties break up the phlegm and help the body to get rid of it.

Bitter foods are very good for anybody who suffers with sinus problems, mucus in the lungs and congestion on the face. Some bitter foods include rhubarb, kale, watercress and celery. Bitter foods can combat chronic congestion in the nose, lungs or face, as well as yeast overgrowth, obesity and skin eruptions. The bitter taste also increases intestinal muscle contraction which helps with the peristalsis movement of the intestines. This is very helpful if one has a sluggish colon, been traveling, or eating junk food, and is constipated.

Pungent

The pungent taste has the function of dispersing, invigorating and promoting circulation. The dispersing quality can help promote circulation or stave off a cold. It is used to break up blood stasis, local

Although raw honey has a sweet taste, it has a pungent, drying effect on the body after digestion. It dries up damp, overweight and mucous conditions but is not useful for dry skin or those who are too thin. Tupelo raw honey is the only honey that diabetics can eat, because it doesn't spike their glucose. When buying honey, make sure that it is "raw" honey. My favorite is raw honey made with ginseng, because the honey tonifies the spleen and the ginseng gives me an extra boost of energy. If you have a weak spleen or pancreas, a teaspoon of raw honey first thing in the morning can be very good to get the digestion going for the day. It will help the pancreas start producing insulin and the enzymes that are necessary to break up the food.

pain, irregular menses, painful menstruation and edema. Examples of pungent foods are ginger, garlic and mint. Their dispersing quality opens the pores and promotes sweating. If you feel a cold coming on, slice up some fresh ginger along with some scallions and drink it; this will help you to sweat and fight the virus.

Tables 10.1, **10.2** and **10.3** categorize the different tastes and foods. You'll notice that many foods fit into more than one category.

Table 10.1 Tastes and Food Categorized

Sour	Bitter	Pungent*	Salty
Lemons	Alfalfa	Radishes	Barley
Limes	Bitter Melons	Scallions	Millet
Pickles	Romaine Lettuce Rye	Turnips	Soy Sauce
Sauerkraut	Radishes	White Pepper	Miso
Sour Apples	Scallions	Leeks	Pickles
Hawthorne Berries	Turnips		Seaweed
Rosehip Chinese	White Pepper		• Kelp
Sour Plums	Vinegar		• Kombu
Vinegar	Celery		• Bladderwrack
Leeks	Lettuce		• Spiru
Apples	Papaya		• Lina
Blackberries	Asparagus		
Grapes	Amaranth		
Mangoes	Quinoa		
Olives			
Raspberries			
Tangerines			
Tomatoes			
Sourdough bread			
Adzuki Beans			

*See Table 10.2 for Pungent Cooling and Warming Foods

Table 10.2 Pungent Cooling and Warming Foods

Pungent Cooling	Pungent Warming
Peppermint	Spearmint
Marjoram	Rosemary
White Pepper	Scallions
Radish	Garlic
Turnips	Entire Onion Family
	Cinnamon Bark and Branches
	Cloves
	Fresh and Dry Ginger
	All Hot Peppers
	Black Pepper
	Cayenne
	Fennel
	Anise
	Dill
	Mustard
	Horseradish
	Basil
	Nutmeg

Table 10.3 Sweet Foods

Fruits	Vegetables	Beans	Nuts	Seeds	Sweeteners
Apricots	Squash • Butternut • Acorn	All Legumes	Almonds	Sesame	Honey
Cherries	Potatoes • Sweet • Yams	Peas	Chestnuts	Sunflower	Molasses
Dates	Corn	Lentils	Coconuts	Walnuts	Barley Malt
Figs	Yellow Peppers				
Peaches					
Pears					
Strawberries					
Grapefruit					

Chapter 11

Acupuncture

The Western concept of well-being is based on the fact that we must have sufficient blood flow to all of our organs and tissues to be healthy. Blood carries all the vital nutrients our cells need to function, heal and fight infection. If our organs don't get enough blood, they can't function properly and will eventually contract some form of disease. Consider the example of a garden hose. If the hose has a kink, the garden doesn't receive water and plants begin to die. The same concept applies to the human body. If qi is blocked, the flow cannot reach our organs and tissues. Acupuncture can help restore the flow and bring the body back to homeostasis.

Acupuncture is based on the idea that health is determined by the balanced flow of qi, or energy, through the entire body.

As we discussed in chapters 2 and 3, qi travels through the body via invisible paths called meridians. Each meridian is connected to a particular vital organ and its job is to bring blood, nutrients and qi to that organ. There are over 1,000 acupuncture pressure points (acupoints) on the meridian system that can be stimulated to enhance the flow of qi. To accomplish this, fine, hair-like needles are inserted into these acupoints. It is the acupuncturist's job to figure out where the blockage is and determine in which acupoint to insert a needle.

Qi can be blocked, sluggish, deficient or exuberant. Any of these issues can eventually cause pain or illness. For example, if your lung qi is weak, you may suffer from asthma; if your knee qi is blocked, you may have pain and arthritis in your knees. Acupuncture addresses illness by finding and repairing blockages and low levels of qi in the body's meridians. Acupuncturists not only look at the specific area that is hurting, but at the specific meridian or organ affected.

Acupuncture can help to bring the body back into balance by toning, sedating or unblocking the channel affected.

It is beneficial to have acupuncture periodically to make sure all the meridians are flowing smoothly. Some of the benefits of acupuncture include:

- Can be implemented simultaneously with other medical treatments or prescriptions
- Strengthens the immune system
- May allow for faster recovery from injuries
- Improves circulation
- Decreases symptoms of stress
- Can alleviate feelings of illness that are physically nonexistent; strengthens ones' overall well-being
- Can alleviate skin problems like acne, rosacea, psoriasis, and eczema
- Has the ability to reduce or cure emotional or psychological disorders
- Can treat:
  - Infertility
  - Digestive disorders
  - Sleep disorders
  - Migraines and headaches
  - Menstrual problems

Though minor, acupuncture does include some risks. These include:
- Minimal bleeding after removal of the needles (3% of patients)
- Bruising around puncture points (2% of patients)
- Dizziness (1% of patients)

Before obtaining treatment, be sure your acupuncturist is highly trained, attended an accredited school and has passed the NCCAOM

(National Certification Commission for Acupuncture and Oriental Medicine) national boards.

> For more information on NCCAOM, visit their web site at http://www.nccaom.org/.

Educational credentials in the US vary widely from a diploma or certificate in acupuncture to a PhD or D.O.M. (Doctor of Oriental Medicine). **Table 11.1** shows the most common criteria. The laws of the various states and the requirements change rapidly, so please check with your local boards.

Table 11.1 **Educational Criteria for Acupuncturists**

Designation	Curriculum
AP-Acupuncture Physician	2-3 years undergraduate + 3 years of graduate study. Must pass the three basic national board exams.
DOM-Doctor of Oriental Medicine	Same as an AP but has also taken another board on Chinese herbs.
PhD	(Only in California so far) 2 more years of study.Entails doing research on a particular area of specialty.

Acupuncture is a good preventative medicine and will ensure you remain in optimal health for many years. The patients I serve are in their 60s and 70s. They are living actively and remain proactive in maintaining their good health. They tell me they have never felt so good and have a lot of energy to enjoy their "golden years".

Chapter 12

Facial Acupuncture

You might have read about facial acupuncture or heard clients talking about it. It is a service that is becoming very popular among the rich and famous. Facial acupuncture is a painless, non-surgical method of reducing signs of the aging process. Though facial acupuncture has sometimes been referred to as an "acupuncture facelift", it is more than a cosmetic procedure. It is a revitalization process designed to help the whole body look and feel younger.

The facial acupuncture treatment is based on principles of traditional Chinese medicine and, as in standard acupuncture, involves the insertion of hair-thin needles into particular areas of the face, ear, neck, hands, trunk, and legs. Specific points are chosen to manipulate the movement of energy in the body according to the individual patient's needs. We customize the treatment to the underlying deficiencies of the body that are contributing to aging and use acupuncture to stimulate blood circulation up to the face. When the needles are inserted into the fine lines of the face, it causes a sort of micro-trauma to the skin causing the skin to produce more protein. This plumps up the skin, reducing the look of fine lines and wrinkles.

Facial acupuncture can erase as many as five to 10 years from the face with results visible after a few treatments. A few other benefits include:
- Fine lines softened
- Deeper wrinkles significantly diminished
- Bags under the eyes reduced
- Jowls firmed

- Puffiness eliminated
- Droopy eyelids lifted
- Double chins minimized

Other likely results include moisturization of the skin, increased local circulation of blood and lymph to the face, increased collagen production, increased muscle tone, tightening of the pores, hormonal balance to help acne and the reduction of stress evident on the face (the line between the eyebrows).

Facial acupuncture is contraindicated for some pituitary disorders, heart disorders, diabetes mellitus, high blood pressure, individuals who have pace makers, or who have a problem with bleeding, bruising or suffer from migraine headaches.

> Facial acupuncture should not be done during pregnancy, a bout with a cold or flu, an allergic attack or an acute herpes outbreak.

Facial acupuncture is usually done in a series of 6 to 12 treatments with the patient receiving a treatment once a week. The procedure takes about an hour and a half to perform and consists of a comprehensive intake (health and lifestyle history), facial cleansing, exfoliation, and acupuncture to the body before moving to the face. The needles stay in for about twenty minutes before being removed. The procedure is followed by a facial massage, mask and moisturizer for the client's particular skin type. After the initial series, the patient usually returns for maintenance treatments every three months, during which time an assessment is done to see if there any new concerns that need to be addressed.

Facial acupuncture has great results, but the patient will see results faster if they follow a good home skin care regime, exercise, and eat a nutritious diet.

Chapter 13

Qigong

The word Qigong (pronounced "chee gong") is a combination of two words: "Qi," the vital energy of the body, and "Gong," which is the practice of self-discipline. Qigong is an exercise technique practiced in China to promote health and well-being. It involves the coordination of breathing patterns, movements and meditation.

The practice of Qigong dates back to 58 A.D. when the Han Emperor of China adopted Buddhism from India. It began as a method for promoting health, longevity and beauty within the royal family, but many of the Qigong practices and Buddhist meditations from India disseminated into Chinese culture as a way to keep everyone healthy and flexible.

Qigong is different from Western exercises like jogging, biking and aerobic exercise; these activities promote strengthening of the body. Qigong, on the other hand, helps strengthen the internal organs and increase the flow of qi throughout the body. If the internal organs are healthy and qi is flowing smoothly, muscle tone and body strength happen naturally.

The practice of Qigong includes many moving exercises. To maintain health and productivity throughout the workday, many Chinese include such exercises in their morning routines. Two of the most popular include the "Five Animal Frolics" and the "Eight Brocades." Hua Tuo, a famous physician who lived between 110 and 207 A.D., developed "Five Animal Frolics" an exercise in which one imitates the actions of apes, bears, birds, deer and tigers. The "Eight Brocades" game was created by an army officer during the Sung dynasty (960-1279 A.D.) who wished to maintain his soldiers' health.

There are many different forms of Qigong, but all incorporate slow movements of the body along with meditation and deep breathing. It is believed that the regular practice of Qigong helps cleanse the body of toxins, restore energy, reduce stress and anxiety, as well as maintain a healthy and active lifestyle. The exercise motions can be done while sitting, standing or moving.

Three important principles to a beneficial Qigong practice are posture, relaxation and a focused mind. Good posture must be maintained at all times and the spine must remain straight. This is accomplished by concentrating on three areas along the spine: the top of the sacrum, behind the heart and the base of the skull. Focusing on these regions and mentally lifting them upward will create good posture, which in turn will allow qi to flow smoothly. This is a wonderful exercise for estheticians who are sitting all day long in their treatment chairs.

The relaxation we are talking about is not just letting the body go limp; it is a way of relaxing the body with a focused mind. This means getting rid of external voices and focusing on what you are doing. Where the mind goes, energy follows. If you are anxious or depressed and concentrate on that, the body's energy will be depleted and you'll become more depressed or anxious. However, if you focus on being calm, relaxed and healthy, your body's energy will respond and your body will be relaxed and healthy. Focus on loving your vibrant, healthy skin and your body will respond

> Before beginning treatment on a client, think about your posture and keeping your spine straight; then mentally pull up from the three areas and take a deep breath. If you maintain good posture, you will not be so tired at the end of the day, and it will be easier to maintain good posture for longer periods of time.

by helping you have beautiful skin. Focus on the fine lines and hyperpigmentation and your body will respond by accentuating those issues. The meditation I am going to describe will help you and your clients visualize the healthy, beautiful skin you desire.

The exercise I am about to describe is a sitting meditation that takes about five to 10 minutes and can be done at any time. The purpose of this meditation is to soften the fine lines and give the face a healthy glow, but the moving exercises also stimulate all the meridians to bring about optimal health and longevity.

Before beginning this exercise, focus your mind on a point called the "Dan Tien." This point is the body's center of gravity and is considered the body's vital energy center. It is located about 4 fingers below the belly button. Concentrate on this area until you feel the energy. Visualize an energy center that begins as a ball and then travels to other parts of the body.

The Qigong Meditation for Facial Rejuvenation

1. Sit comfortably in a chair with your legs shoulder-length apart. Make sure that your spine is straight. Loosely rest your hands in your lap.

2. Breathing should be relaxed and even. This might require you to focus on your breath to remove distractions from your mind so you can be present in the moment.

3. Place both your hands on your "Dan Tien" and focus your mind on this point until you feel energy or until the palms of your hands are warm.

4. In your mind, create a beautiful ball of energy. It can be any color that you want. Most people visualize a ball of red or white energy.

5. Send the energy ball up the Ren channel, which runs

The ren channel is responsible for the yin aspect of the body, while the du is responsible for the yang aspect. By sending the energy ball up and down these two channels, you are stimulating the yin and yang of the body.

up the center of the body, to the top of the head and then down the Du channel, which runs down the spinal column, and return it to the Dan Tien. Do this about five times.

6. Now imagine that the pores of your skin are opening up and breathing in healthy qi and at the same time releasing toxins out of the skin. Do this for five breaths while both hands are still holding the energy ball at the Dan Tien.

7. Now send the energy ball up the middle of your body again, but this time when it reaches the chin, the ball will split into two smaller balls of energy that are big enough to be held in the palms of your hands.

8. Next, imagine massaging your forehead and temporal area, and picture all the lines fading away. Imagine massaging your cheek area and the redness disappearing; visualize massaging your mouth area and the fine lines disappearing; and then to the chin to tone and strengthen your jaw line. Go up and down the nasal labial groove to soften the line there. Massage any area that concerns you and send the healing energy into that area to resolve the issue. Then visualize what it would look like if it were perfect.

9. Go back to your chin with both energy balls and make one energy ball that travels down the Ren to the Dan Tien. Hold the energy ball at the Dan Tien until you visualize it entering your body, sending the healing energy all through your body.

10. Take three deep breaths and focus on three things about your face that please you. It could be your smile, beautiful eyes, dimples or freckles. Concentrate on them and give thanks.

Chapter 14

Facial Acupressure Massage

This particular acupressure massage technique is one that I teach my clients. I suggest using this massage technique at home once a day to help soften fine lines and firm up the chin and jaw area. It will also provide a sense of tranquility and peace.

There are 21 acupressure points that will be massaged one at a time; 18 are located on the face, one on the neck, one on the hand, and one on the elbow. It will take about 15 minutes to do the whole massage. At each point, massage 20 times in a clockwise direction with the finger(s) indicated. The massage can be done while washing the face in the morning or evening, or at any time during the day. After the points have been memorized, a mirror will not be needed and it can even be done while walking on the treadmill or watching television.

To prepare:
1. Wash hands
2. Sit in a relaxed position with a mirror
3. Relax the neck to avoid putting too much pressure on the neck muscles

Most of the following points are points that are located on different meridians along the face. There are 2 points that are not located on a

If you become tired during the massage, stop, shake out your hands, take a few deep breaths and continue.

meridian. Though they are not located on a meridian, massaging them has been found to be beneficial to the skin and face.

We will begin on meridian points located on the forehead so we can direct the qi and blood flow up to the face. We will then work our way down to the neck, hand and, lastly, to the elbow.

The massage

1. Gallbladder 15

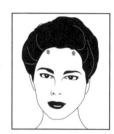

Location:
Located on the forehead within the anterior hairline, directly above the pupil when the eyes are looking straight ahead.

Procedure:
Use your index fingers and massage both sides at the same time.

Applications:
- Relieving headaches
- Softening the lines across the forehead

2. Gallbladder 14

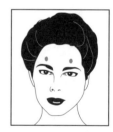

Location:
Located on the forehead, one inch directly above the pupil when the eye is looking straight ahead.

Procedure:
Use your index fingers and massage both sides at the same time.

Applications:
- Sagging eyelids
- Headaches
- Twitching of the eyelids

3. Yintang

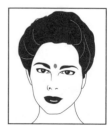

Location:
Located between the eyebrows, at the upper border of the nose.

Procedure:

Use your index finger to massage this point.

Applications:

- Calming the client
- Softening the fine lines between the eyebrows
- Treating sinuses
- Relieving frontal headache

4. Bladder 2

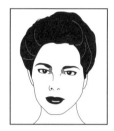

Location:

Located in the inner canthus of the eye, in the depression on the eyebrow.

Procedure:

Use your thumb to massage this point.

Applications:

- Sagging eyebrows
- Sinus headaches
- Sneezing
- Stuffy nose

5. Yuyao (Extra Point)

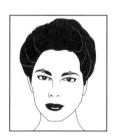

Location:

Located in the center of the eyebrow.

Procedure:

Use your index finger to massage. Push up on the eyebrow and massage where the eyebrow would have been.

Applications:

- Sagging eyelids
- Twitching of the eyelid
- Frontal headache

6. Triple Heater 23

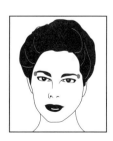

Location:

Located at the outer end of the eyebrow.

Procedure:

Use your index finger to massage this point.

Applications:

- Softening crow's feet
- Stopping eye twitches
- Relieving temporal headaches

7. Gallbladder 1

Location:

Located on the outer lower side of the eye, in the outer orbital ridge.

Procedure:

Use your index finger to massage this point.

Applications:

- Softening crow's feet
- Treating dark circles under the eyes

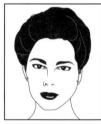

8. Front and Back sides of the Ears

Procedure:

Use two fingers to massage this area; your index finger massages the back of the ear and the middle finger massages the front. Go up and down with the fingers to stimulate this acupressure point.

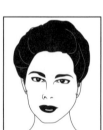

Applications:

- Stimulates lymph fluid to the face and ear areas
- Treats ringing in the ears
- Addresses Temporomandibular joint diseases and disorders (TMJD's)
- Relieves temporal headaches

9. Stomach 2

Location:

Located one-half inch directly below the eye when the pupil is looking straight head.

Procedure:

Use your index finger to massage this point, but be very gentle with the thin skin.

Applications:

- Skin color
- Puffiness under the eyes
- Dark circles under the eyes
- Sinus congestion

10. Stomach 3

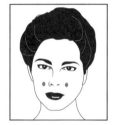

Location:

Located directly below Stomach 2 at the level of the lower border of the nose in the nasal labial groove.

Procedure:

Use your index and middle fingers to massage this point; get under the cheekbone.

Applications:

- Reducing facial swelling
- Helping to define the cheek area
- Treating sinuses
- Relieving toothaches

11. Du 26

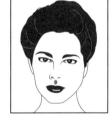

Location:

Located directly above the lips in the middle of the philtrum (vertical groove in the upper lip).

Procedure:

Use your index finger to massage this point.

Applications:

- Lines around the mouth
- Loss of consciousness
- Dizziness and nausea
- Back spasms (pinch this point to treat spasms)

12. Stomach 4

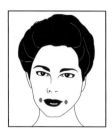

Location:

Located on the sides of the mouth in the nasal labial groove.

Procedure:

Use two fingers to massage this point. One finger is on the point and the other finger is a little farther out than the nasal labial groove.

Applications:

- Treat lines around the mouth
- Correct deviation of the mouth
- Soften the nasal labial groove
- Relieves toothaches

13. Ren 24

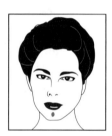

Location:

Located directly below the mouth in the middle of the chin.

Procedure:

Use your index finger to massage this point.

Applications:

- Hormonal breakouts
- Hormonal imbalances
- Grinding of teeth
- Gums of clients with tooth pain
- Dry mouth or excessive salivation

14. Small Intestine 18

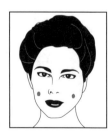

Location:

Located directly below the outer canthus of the eye in the cheek hollow.

Procedure:

Use your index finger to massage this point.

Applications:
- Treats facial swelling
- Treats TMJD's
- Alleviates toothaches
- Helps with facial contour

15. Stomach 7

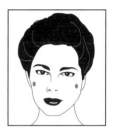

Location:
Located at the lower border of the cheek bone in the depression at the front of the ear.

Procedure:
Use your index finger to massage it.

Applications:
- Treats TMJD's
- Relieves earaches
- Relieves toothaches
- Treats lockjaw
- Treats ear disorders

16. Jaw Line

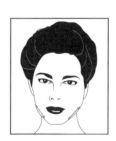

Location:
This area is located right below the jaw.

Procedure:
Use all fingers to massage the jaw line area.

Applications:
- Drooping jowls
- Chicken neck
- Slacking of the neck

17. Ren 23

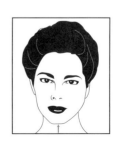

Location:
Located directly under the chin.

Procedure:
Use index finger to massage this point.

Applications:
- Benefits the tongue
- Addresses excessive or insufficient saliva in the mouth
- Treats chicken neck

18. Stomach 9

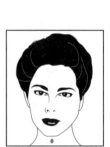

Location:

Located level with the Adam's apple, on the anterior border of the Sternocleidomastoid Muscle (SCM).

Procedure:

Use index finger and massage with up and down movements.

Applications:
- Regulating the thyroid
- Relieving sore throats
- Treating indigestion
- Addressing difficulty in swallowing
- Eliminating hiccups

19. Ren 22

Location:

Located just below the hollow of the lower border of the neck.

Procedure:

Use index finger to massage this point.

Applications:
- Hiccups
- Indigestion
- Coughing
- Difficulty swallowing
- Dry throat

20. Large Intestine 4

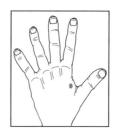

Location:

Located on the back of the hand between the thumb and the index finger, in the middle of the web. This point is the master point for the face.

Procedure:

Massage each hand one at a time using the thumb and index finger.

Applications:

- Relieves headaches
- Relieves toothaches
- Relieves nasal congestion
- Relieves nose bleeds

Do not massage the Large Intestine 4 point if you are pregnant!

21. Large Intestine 11

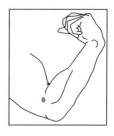

Location:

Located in the outer crease of the elbow when the elbow is bent.

Procedure:

Use the thumb to massage this point one elbow at a time.

Applications:

- Psoriasis
- Eczema
- Fevers
- Hives
- Relieves sore throats
- Relieves toothaches

Take a few deep breaths and shake out the arms.

After the 15-minute massage, the qi and blood will be flowing freely around the face, giving it a fresh, healthy glow.

Chapter 15

Soups for the Skin

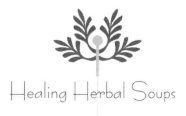

Healing Herbal Soups

Soups are excellent for nourishing the skin and bringing wonderful nutrients into the body. The following recipes address common skin conditions, though they are beneficial to those without skin concerns as well. The soups are divided into categories by the conditions that can be improved by eating them.

Most soups are made from a vegetable, beef or chicken stock. You can purchase these in a can at the grocery store, but be aware some are very salty. If you are in a pinch and don't have the time to make a stock, make sure to buy one that states "low sodium" or "organic."

Frozen stock can be kept in the freezer for up to three months. Make sure you label each stock carefully for easy identification later.

The soups in this chapter can be purchased online at *www.healingherbalsoups.com*

Stock Recipes

Vegetable Stock—makes 10 cups

Ingredients

    1 tablespoon olive oil
    1 large onion, quartered
    2 cups carrots, chopped
    2 celery stocks, chopped thinly
    ½ cup scallions, chopped
    6 garlic gloves, smashed
    8 parsley sprigs with stems
    ½ teaspoon of died thyme
    1 sprig fresh rosemary
    2 bay leaves
    1 teaspoon sea salt
    Freshly ground pepper to taste
    15 cups cold water

Directions

1. Put the olive oil in the stockpot. Add the first four ingredients and cook. Stir frequently over medium heat for 10 minutes or until lightly brown. Add the rest of the ingredients.
2. Bring to a boil; reduce the heat and simmer slowly, partially covered. Cook the stock at least 30 minutes at a simmer, strain it and add it to your soup. It can also be frozen and pulled out whenever you want to make a soup with a vegetable stock.

Chicken Stock—makes 10 cups

Ingredients

    3 pounds whole chicken
    2 onions cut into quarters
    1 tablespoon olive oil
    2 carrots chopped
    2 celery stalks, chopped
    8 parsley sprigs
    1 teaspoon dried thyme
    2 bay leaves
    10 black peppercorns, lightly crushed
    16 cups cold water

Directions

1. Put the olive oil on the bottom of the stockpot, add the chicken and onion and cook until light brown.
2. Add all other ingredients, bring to a boil and simmer for 3 hours with the lid partly open. The chicken should be so tender it falls off the bone.
3. When the mixture is cold, remove the layer of fat on the top; it is now ready to be added to your soup or frozen.
4. The fat can be saved and used to sauté vegetables or other items.
5. Remove the chicken from the bones and save for use in the soup or other items.

Beef Stock—makes 10 cups

This stock is very time consuming to make, but if your client has been very sick or lost a lot of blood, they will benefit from all the nutrients in the homemade stock. Pre-made beef broth can be purchased, but again beware of the sodium content. I have had a hard time finding soup bones from a regular grocery store. You might have to go to a butcher and ask them to special order them for you.

Ingredients

5 pounds of beef bones.
2 onions, quartered with skin on
2 carrots, chopped with skin on
2 celery stocks, chopped
2 tomatoes, coarsely chopped
8 parsley sprigs with stems
1 teaspoon thyme
2 bay leaves
1 tablespoon course black pepper
8 cups cold water

> You can go to the butcher and ask for the knuckle bones. Request he cut the bones into 2 ½ inch pieces to make a beef stock.

Directions

1. Preheat the oven to 450° F, put the bones in a roasting pan or casserole dish, and roast the bones for about 30 minutes until they start to brown.
2. Add the onions, carrots, celery and tomatoes; roast for another 30 minutes; stir occasionally until the bones are well-browned.
3. Transfer the bones and the roasted vegetables to a stockpot. Add the water and remaining ingredients.
4. Bring the stock to a boil and let it simmer for 12 hours partly covered. The bones and vegetables should always maintain original water level throughout the cooking process, so add more water when necessary.
5. Strain the stock through a colander and refrigerate. Remove the fat off the top before using or freezing.
6. The natural fats can be used for sautéing or cooking, if desired.

Soup Recipes

The following soup recipes were written by my husband Philip Guilbeault. He has been an executive chef for over forty years and helped me put my herbal knowledge into recipes people can drink. I couldn't have written this chapter without his expertise and support.

I am partial to soups because of all their fresh nutrients and many benefits. Many people have a spleen-pancreas deficiency because they are not breaking down their food enough for nutrients to be absorbed. Soups are already partially broken down; therefore they are very easy on the digestive track and considered a "comfort food." They can be consumed as a beverage during the day or as a complete meal.

Some of the ingredients used in these soups are Chinese herbs that can be purchased online or at most Asian grocery markets. If you can't find the Chinese herbs, you will still benefit a great deal from other ingredients that can be purchased at most grocery stores. These recipes are for you to try and tweak for your taste or condition.

Soups for Acne or Blemished Skin

The following soups are designed to help clients that have occasional breakouts, premenstrual breakouts or chronic acne. They are also good for cleansing the system if you've been consuming an excess of junk food or alcohol.

Liver Tonic (Detox Soup for Acne)

Benefits

This soup can be drank every day for lunch or dinner to alleviate acne or stressed-out skin. The client should drink this until the acne starts to get better or the formation of new papules and pustules has ceased. This is also a great soup to drink for about seven days in the spring to help cleanse the liver. Do not eat heavy, rich foods, dairy, sugar, alcohol or processed foods because they will inhibit the cleansing of the liver.

Ingredients

2 tablespoons olive oil
1 large onion, chopped
5 garlic cloves, chopped
8 fresh mint leaves
1 cup fresh lotus root, sliced
1 cup bitter melon, cut into rings
1 cup chopped parsley
2 handfuls watercress
2 cups dandelion greens

1 cup burdock root, sliced
3 cups beet greens
1 or 2 handfuls of odd greens (carrot or radish tops)
½ cup fennel seeds
Sea salt and pepper to taste
Fresh lemon juice or vinegar to taste

Directions

1. Warm the oil in a wide soup pot. Add the onions and garlic and cook over medium heat for several minutes until the onions are transparent, and then add the rest of the ingredients. Season with 1½ teaspoons of salt. Cook over medium heat for about five minutes or until the greens have collapsed and turn every few minutes.
2. Once the greens have wilted, add two quarts of water. Bring to a boil and simmer for 25 minutes. Cool briefly and then puree. Either leave the soup with some texture or make it smooth.
3. Taste for salt, season with pepper and add the lemon juice or vinegar.

Liver-Soothing and Blood-Tonifying Soup

Benefits

This tonic is great when acne flares up and the infection has spread. The charred red radicchio is added to cool the blood and promotes circulation of new blood up to the face to stop the infection from spreading.

This soup is also good for clients who suffer from head-aches on the sides of the head or from eczema around the ears. They should have a bowl of soup for one week or until the infection has stopped spreading. As with any other tonic for the liver, the client should not drink alcohol or eat heavy or processed foods, dairy or sweets while trying to get the infection under control.

Another suggestion for acne clients: before reaching for a cup of coffee or tea, drink a cup of hot lemon water first thing in the morning. The lemon's sour taste will wake up the liver and help it secrete the old bile that has been stored in the gall-bladder all night.

Ingredients

2 tablespoons olive oil

2 shallots, finely chopped

3 garlic cloves, crushed

5 leeks, chopped (make sure to cut them lengthwise and rinse with cold water to remove sand before chopping)

2 cups zucchini, chopped

1 cup bitter melon, cut into rings

5 cups water

2 cups dandelion greens

1 cup chervil, chopped

1 cup fresh parsley, chopped

½ cup fresh mint, chopped

1 round lettuce, separated into leaves

4 cups vegetable stock

2 large heads red radicchios, cut into wedges
Sea salt and ground pepper

Directions

1. Put the olive oil, shallots and garlic into a cold soup pan and cook for two to three minutes until the shallots and garlic are softened but not browned.
2. Add the leeks, bitter melon and zucchini with enough vegetable stock to cover the vegetables; put a lid on the pan and cook for 15 minutes.
3. Add the fresh herbs and lettuce. Cook for about three minutes or until wilted.
4. Cut the radicchios into quarters and brush with olive oil. Heat the grill or frying pan until very hot and add the radicchios. Cook the radicchios for 1 minute on each side until slightly charred and add to the soup.
5. Pour the remaining vegetable stock and simmer for 15 minutes. Cool the soup slightly, and then run it through a food processor or blender until smooth. Return the soup to the rinsed pan and season well.

Soups for Asphyxiated Skin

For those with an abundance of whiteheads and/or blackheads but no redness or pustules, this type of skin requires an invigorated spleen-pancreas and increased blood circulation. The following two soups will invigorate the qi and move blood to the face. This will bring new oxygen and lymph fluid into the face, which will help clear out congestion and produce a radiant look. All three of the following soups can be made in a big pot and drank once a day for about 10 days. I recommend eating this soup for an evening meal so that it won't hinder digestion overnight.

Spleen-Pancreas Deficiency Soup (Rev-up the Metabolism Soup)

Benefits

We use this soup to treat sagging skin, droopy eyelids, lines around the mouth and a pale, sallow complexion. It is also great for anybody who is tired and has a weak digestion. The dried astralagus (Huang Qi) can be purchased at any Asian grocery store. It looks like sliced white bark.

Ingredients

½ cup olive oil
3 cups butternut squash, peeled, seeded and cubed
2 carrots, cut into thick rounds
1 rutabaga, peeled and cut into ½ inch cubes
1 onion, quartered
5 garlic cloves, peeled
½ a ginger root, peeled and cubed
10 sticks dried astralagus (Huang Qi)
6 sticks Poria (Fu Ling)
3 bay leaves
1 tablespoon nutmeg
2 teaspoons cinnamon
10 cups chicken stock
Salt and pepper to season
Sour cream, to serve on top

> To avoid burning, you might want to wear plastic gloves when you are seeding and chopping the chili.

Directions

1. Preheat oven to 400° F
2. Pour the olive oil into a large bowl, add the prepared vegetables and toss thoroughly with a spoon until they are coated with oil.
3. Spread the vegetables on a large baking sheet.
4. Roast the vegetables for about 50 minutes until tender, turning them occasionally to make sure they brown evenly. Remove from the oven and transfer to a large pot.
5. Pour the stock into the pot and bring to a boil. Reduce the heat, add the cinnamon and nutmeg, season to taste and then simmer for 10 minutes. Transfer the soup to a food processor or hand blender and mix for a few minutes until it is thick and smooth.
6. Return the soup to the pot to heat through. Season and serve.

Skin Lifting Soup

Benefits

This is another great soup to help sagging skin. It is also beneficial for droopy eyelids and jowls, and for removing lines around the mouth.

Ingredients

6 tablespoons olive oil
4 pounds pumpkin
2 pounds cubed sweet potatoes
2 onions, chopped
3 garlic cloves, chopped
½ cup fresh ginger, grated
15 pieces dried astralagus (Huang Qi)
1 teaspoon cardamom pods
1 teaspoon nutmeg
2 teaspoons cinnamon
10 cups chicken stock
Sea salt and pepper to taste
1 teaspoon toasted black sesame seeds for garnish

Directions

1. Heat 4 tablespoons of oil in a large pan, add the onions, garlic and ginger and cook for 4 to 5 minutes. Add the pumpkin, sweet potatoes, coriander, cinnamon and nutmeg and cook for two minutes. Pour in the chicken stock and astralagus. Bring to a boil, reduce the heat and simmer for 50 minutes, or until all the ingredients are soft.

2. Cool the soup lightly and then puree it in a food processor or blender until smooth. Return the soup to the pan to reheat and season well. Ladle the soup and garnish with some toasted black sesame seeds.

Lung-and Spleen-Pancreas-Warming Soup

Benefits

The main ingredient in this soup is parsnip, a white herb that helps the lung. The lungs are in charge of the pores. Therefore, this soup warms up the spleen-pancreas to remove congestion from the pores. It doesn't push it out; it just warms up sebum so it doesn't stay congested in the pore.

Ingredients

½ cup olive oil

1 onion, chopped

2 garlic cloves, crushed

1 green chili, seeded and finely chopped

2 tablespoons grated fresh ginger

5 pieces cinnamon bark

2 cups parsnips, cubed

2 cups cauliflower

1 cup green apples, chopped

1 teaspoon cumin seeds

1 teaspoon coriander

2 teaspoons nutmeg

15 sticks astralagus (Huang Qi)

10 sticks poria (Fu Ling)

1 teaspoon curry

5 cups water

Juice of one lime

Salt and black pepper to taste

Handful of fresh cilantro, chopped for garnish

Directions

1. Heat the oil in a large pot and add the onions, ginger, garlic and chili. Cook for four to five minutes, until the onion is soft or lightly brown. Add the parsnips and cauliflower and cook for two to three minutes. Sprinkle with cumin seeds, coriander, nutmeg, cinnamon and curry, and cook for one minute, stirring occasionally.

2. Add the green apples, season well and bring back to boil. Reduce the heat and simmer for 15 minutes, until all vegetables are soft.

3. Cook the soup slightly, then mix it in a food processor or blender until smooth and return it to the pot; stir in the lime juice.

4. Ladle the soup into bowls and garnish with the fresh cilantro.

You might want to wear plastic gloves when you are seeding and chopping the chili

Soups that Nourish the Liver

The next two soups (Liver Yin-Nourishing and Liver Blood-Nourishing) are great for helping to diminish fine lines, especially around the eyes. These soups are great for nourishing the liver blood. It is beneficial to consume this soup in more of a cyclic pattern. I recommend a client have a bowl once a day for a week and then take a week off.

This soup should be consumed if a client's eye area feels tired, if they feel they are showing signs of aging or if they have recently undergone Botox as this soup will help the results last longer and give the face a healthy glow.

Both soups contain very tasty Chinese herbs. One of the ingredients, wolfberries, can be put in a pot of hot water and consumed as a beverage; eating the moist berries can also be helpful, as it will nourish the liver and kidney yin while also helping the lung yin. When a client has a lung yin deficiency, they will likely experience a dry cough and throat; this soup is also healthful for such ailments.

Liver Yin-Nourishing Soup

Benefits

This soup can be served hot or cold if your client is having hot flashes and/or has a very red face.

Ingredients

½ cup olive oil
1 cup onion, chopped
1 cup yellow chrysanthemum flowers
8 cooked beets, diced
2 cups plum tomatoes, chopped
1 white cabbage, shredded
10 cups vegetable stock
1 tablespoon sugar
1 tablespoon cider vinegar
1 tablespoon chopped fresh dill
25 wolfberries
25 red jujubes
Salt and pepper to taste

Directions

1. Put the onion, diced beets, tomatoes, cabbage and vegetable stock in a large pot. Bring to a boil, reduce heat and simmer for 30 minutes or until the beets are tender.
2. Add the sugar, wolfberries, jujubes, chrysanthemum flowers and vinegar to the soup and cook for 10 minutes. Taste for a good sweet-sour balance.
3. Stir in the chopped dill and ladle into warm bowls immediately. Garnish with more dill.

No salt or pepper should be added to this soup at any time, not even when serving.

Liver Blood-Nourishing Soup (Recovery Soup)

Benefits

Here is another soup helpful to the eye area. It will also nourish the blood, which will benefit the entire face. I have added a Chinese herb called "He Shou Wu" to this soup. He Shou Wu means "black hair" in Chinese. Many of the Chinese drink it as a tea when their hair starts to turn gray. It is a wonderful herb that tonifies the liver and kidney yin. It is used here for the eye area, but is also very good for treating uterine bleeding, irregular menses, infertility and aging. The taste is very bland, but it works very well with the wolfberries and jujubes to nourish the liver, which in turn nourishes the eye area. The other herb that has been added to this soup is prepared licorice. Licorice is a wonderful adrenal tonic with the capability of entering all 12 meridians; it is a wonderful herb for leg and abdominal cramps and it softens the bitter taste of other herbs.

Ingredients

4 ounces olive oil

12 ounces onions, chopped

4 ounces celery stalk, chopped

3 bay leaves

1 pound well-washed beet greens (optional: use red Swiss chard instead)

20 ounces dry weight leeks (washed well, cut into rounds)

8 ounces carrots, chopped

4 ounces red pepper, peeled, seeded and diced

22 ounces small beets, cut into wedges

1 pound fresh plum tomatoes, diced

2 ounces minced garlic

2 ounces brown sugar

1 ounce fresh basil

4 ounces wolfberries (Gou Qi Zi)

2 ounces red Chinese dates (Da Zao)

3 ounces prepared polygonum (He Shou Wu)

½ ounce whole anise (Ba Jiao)

1 ounce lemon juice

1 pound red lentils

5 quarts of water

Directions

1. Warm oil in a 10 quart pot and add the first 7 ingredients. Cook on low for 15 minutes.
2. Add remaining ingredients, except water, and cook on low for 15 more minutes.
3. Add water and simmer until beets are softened. Do not let water level drop from original point.
4. Let soup cool, then puree on low.

Soups for Menopausal Skin

As your female client experiences the emotional and physical stresses of menopause, she will go through mood swings and insomnia. At the same time, her skin may become drier, thinner, redder and more sensitive due to depletion of estrogen.

To help with the dryness of the skin, most women should consume essential oils. The essential oil 6, "Evening Primrose", is full of estrogen and can be very healing to dry skin.

The Yin-Nourishing Soup

Benefits

This soup is great for yin deficient skin that is dry, thin and starting to show signs of aging. The main ingredient is tofu, which is a wonderful source of estrogen. It also has lily bulbs and lotus root, both of which are very nourishing to the yin.

Some of the ingredients can only be found in an Asian grocery store, but most cities now have a wide variety of Asian markets. The ingredients in this soup can be found in Thai, Chinese, Vietnamese and Korean markets.

Ingredients

½ cup peanut oil

12 ounces firm tofu, cut into small bite-size pieces

10 lily bulbs (Bai He)

2 cups lotus root, sliced

8 star anise

10 cups vegetable stock

1 tablespoon fresh mint

Grated rind 1 kaffir lime

3 kaffir lime leaves, shredded

3 red chilies, seeded and shredded

2 tablespoons lemongrass stalks, finely chopped

2 cups shiitake mushrooms, thinly sliced

1 cup (prepared) He Shou Wu

1 cup alfalfa sprouts

3 tablespoons lime juice

1 teaspoon sugar

1 cup mung beans

1 cup bitter melon, cubed

Sea salt and pepper to taste

Directions

1. Heat the oil in a wok and fry the tofu for four to five minutes or until golden, turning occasionally to brown on all sides. Use a slotted spoon to remove the tofu and set aside. Drain the oil from the wok into a big soup pot.
2. Add the vegetable stock, mint, kaffir lime rind, lime leaves, 2/3 of star anise, lotus root, mung beans and lemongrass to the pan. Bring to a boil and simmer for 20 minutes.
3. Strain the stock into a clean pan; stir in the shiitake mushrooms, He Shou Wu, lily bulbs, spring onions, lime juice and sugar. Simmer for three minutes, add the fried tofu and heat through for five minutes. Mix in the alfalfa sprouts and season to taste. Ladle it into bowls and serve.

Before Surgery Soups

The next two soups (Pre-Surgery and Harmonizing) are excellent for clients about to undergo surgery. They help build up immunity, stimulate the blood flow and aid in the healing process.

Pre-Surgery Soup

Benefits

The mushrooms in this soup are dark, therefore very nourishing to the kidneys; the sour taste stimulates the liver to be in harmony.

Ingredients

1 ounce dried wood ears
20 fresh shiitake mushrooms
10 ounces tofu
1 cup sliced, drained bamboo shoots
10 pieces dried astralagus (Huang Qi)
1 cup He Shou Wu
½ cup licorice
5 cups vegetable stock

4 tablespoons rice vinegar
2 tablespoons sugar
2 tablespoons light soy sauce
1 tablespoon fresh ginger
Sea salt and pepper to taste
2 tablespoons cold water
4 scallions, cut into fine
    rings for garnish

Directions

1. Soak the wood ears and black mushrooms in hot water for 30 minutes or until soft. Drain and chop the ears. Save the water and use it as part of the liquid for the soup.
2. Remove and discard the stalks from the shiitake mushrooms. Cut the caps into thin strips.
3. Cut the tofu into ½ inch cubes and finely shred the bamboo shoots.
4. Place the vegetable stock, mushrooms, tofu, bamboo shoots, astralagus and wood ears in a large pan. Bring the stock to a boil, lower the heat and simmer for about five minutes.
5. Stir in the sugar, He Shou Wu, licorice, vinegar, soy sauce, salt and pepper.
6. Ladle the soup into bowls and garnish with the scallions.

Harmonizing Soup

Benefits

This soup contains lamb, which is very warming to the body. The chick peas are white in color, and therefore help the lungs. Because they are shaped like a heart, they also help promote circulation. The various colors of vegetables benefit all the body's organs.

Ingredients

1 cup chick peas, soaked overnight	8 cups beef stock
3 tablespoons olive oil	2 potatoes, cubed
10 garlic gloves, chopped	1 zucchini, cubed
2 onions, chopped	8 tomatoes, diced
2 parsnips, sliced	½ cup brown or green lentils
3 carrots, sliced	1 pound lamb, cubed
2 teaspoons cumin	2 bay leaves
1 teaspoon turmeric	1 bunch fresh cilantro, chopped
2 tablespoons chopped fresh ginger root	1 cup brown rice
	1 lemon, cut into wedges for garnish

Directions

1. Preheat the oven 250° F. Drain the chick peas.
2. Heat the oil in a large flame-proof casserole dish; add onions, garlic, carrots, cumin, turmeric, parsnips and ginger; cook for two to three minutes. Add the chickpeas, stock, potatoes, zucchini tomatoes, lentils, bay leaves, lamb and cilantro. Cover and cook in the oven for three hours.
3. Cook the brown rice in a pot on the stove while the soup is cooking.
4. Remove the soup from the oven and ladle into a bowl with two scoops of rice. Serve with a lemon wedge.

After Surgery Soups

Soups great for after surgery are those that move and nourish blood as well as help remove stagnation (a bruise is just stagnant blood that is not moving). The main herb to help move the blood is called "Salvia" (Dan Shen). We have also added some dispersing foods to break up the bruises and some blood nourishing foods to bring new blood and oxygen to the wound so it will heal quickly. After surgery, eat foods that are red in color, because they will nourish the heart and improve the circulation of newly oxygenated blood.

Post-Surgery Soup

Benefits

This soup can be drank once or twice a day for about two weeks while recovering from surgery; it will help with bruising and swelling. If the swelling is the primary problem, the Post-Surgery Swollen soup is great to bring the swelling down. Your client can even drink the first soup one day and then the second soup the next day, or one soup at lunch and the other later in the day.

Ingredients

1 cup salvia (Dan Sheen)	½ cup licorice
3 tablespoons olive oil	3 garlic cloves, crushed
3 red bell peppers, seeded and halved	2 pounds ripe, heirloom tomatoes
1cup onion, chopped	1 cup red wine
1 cup red jujubes	6 cups vegetable stock
½ cup plain gelatin	Sea salt and black pepper to taste
½ cup He Shout Wu	1 cup alfalfa sprouts for garnish

Directions

1. Cut each half pepper into quarters and seed. Place skin-side-up on a broiler rack and cook until the skins have charred. Transfer to a bowl and cover with a plate.

2. Heat the oil in a large pan. Add the onions and garlic and cook until lightly brown. Meanwhile, remove the skin from the peppers and roughly chop them. Cut the tomatoes into chunks.

3. Add the peppers and tomatoes to the pan, then cover and cook gently for 10 minutes. Add the red wine, salvia, He Shout Woo, gelatin, and licorice. Cook for another five minutes; then add the stock, salt and pepper and simmer for 20 minutes.

4. Mix the soup in a blender or food processor until smooth. Pour the soup into a container and let it cool before putting it in the refrigerator. Serve the soup cold, garnished with the alfalfa sprouts, which help break up bruises. Celery and asparagus both have dispersing qualities; they can be used as an ingredient in the soup or simply as a garnish.

Post-Surgery Swollen Soup

Ingredients

2 teaspoons olive oil
1 cup onion, chopped
2 cups leeks, sliced
5 cups celery, chopped
1 cup mung beans
1 cup alfalfa sprouts
6 sticks poria (Fu Ling)
10 sticks salvia (Dan Sheen)
8 cups vegetable stock
2 tablespoons chopped fresh chervil
2 tablespoons fennel seeds
1 tablespoon mustard seeds
2 tablespoons celery seeds
½ cup chopped parsley
Sea salt and pepper to taste

Directions

1. Heat the oil in a large pan. Add the onion, leeks and celery; cover and cook gently for about 5 minutes, stirring occasionally.
2. Add mung beans, sprouts, Fu Ling, Dan Shen and stock. Simmer for 30 minutes.
3. Add remaining ingredients and simmer for another 15 minutes.
4. Cool before processing into a smooth consistency.

Miscellaneous Soups

Fragile Capillary Soup

Benefits

This soup will alleviate redness and strengthen the capillaries. It will not alleviate the capillaries that are already distended, but it will strengthen the capillary membranes. The idea is to get rid of the stagnation with green cooling vegetables, as well as red vegetables like tomatoes, to stimulate circulation in a stagnated area. The tomatoes also are very high in bioflavonoid. Bioflavonoid helps strengthen the capillary membranes so they stop distending.

Ingredients

3 tablespoons grape seed oil
2 cups sliced leeks, well-cleaned
3 ounces arugula leaves
2 ounces dandelion greens
10 ounces heirloom tomatoes, quartered
10 ounces plum tomatoes, quartered
10 ounces vine ripped tomatoes, quartered
2 ounces licorice root
4 ounces white radish
10 pieces salvia root
4 cups vegetable stock
1 cup Hawthorne berries
Sea salt and pepper to taste

Directions

1. In a thick-bottomed pan, heat oil and add leeks, arugula and dandelion greens. Simmer lightly for three minutes.
2. Add all remaining ingredients except salt and pepper. Bring to a boil and simmer for 40 minutes.
3. Cool the soup and then puree it in a food processor. Strain through a course strainer and push out as much pulp as possible.
4. Chill in the refrigerator for at least four hours.
5. Ladle into a bowl and add a few ice cubes (for a face that is very red).

Skin Discoloration Soup

Benefits

This soup helps with discoloration on the face. The main ingredients are white radish (Daikon), winter melon and Chinese yams. These three ingredients help to fade hyperpigmentation; however, your clients should also be using a natural, topical skin bleaching agent like Kodiak acid, Japanese mulberry, licorice or vitamin C. Additionally, they always wear sunscreen but avoid the sun as much as possible.

Ingredients

3 tablespoons grape seed oil

1 cup diced onion

3 garlic cloves, diced

2 cups sliced white radish

3 cups wintermelon, cubed

2 Chinese yams, skinned and cut into cubes

1 cup wolfberries (Gou Qi Zi)

1 bunch Bok Choy

1 cup mung beans

8 cups vegetable stock

Directions

1. Heat the oil in a large stock pot. Add the onion and garlic and let them cook for about five minutes or until they turn light brown.
2. Add the rest of the ingredients and bring to a boil. Lower the heat to a simmer and cook for about 30 minutes.
3. Ladle into bowls. You can serve it over pearl barley or brown rice.

The soups recommended in this chapter are just a few examples that will help nourish the body and skin. All are very nutritious, but should be accompanied with an herbal remedy. The herbs are powerful in helping resolve the internal deficiencies or excesses. And remember, the more colors you add to your dishes, the more the body and organs will be nourished internally.

Bibliography

Beinfield, Harriet, and Efrem Korngold. *Between Heaven and Earth: A Guide to Chinese Medicine.* New York: Ballantine, 1991.

Bensky, Dan, and Andrew Gamble. *Chinese Herbal Medicine: Materia Medica.* Seattle: Eastland, 1986.

Deadman, Peter, Mazin, Al-Khafaji, and Kevin Baker. *A Manual of Acupuncture.* Hove: Journal of Chinese Medicine Publications, 2001.

Hay, Louise L. *You Can Heal Your Life.* Carlsbad: Hay House, 1984.

Hicks, Angela. *Thorsons Principles of Chinese Medicine.* San Fransisco: Thorsons Publishers, 1996.

Huang, Li Chun. *Auricular Medicine: The New Era of Medicine and Healing.* Orlando: Auricular International Research and Training Center, 2005.

Jwing-Ming,Yang. *The Root of Chinese Qigong: Secrets for Health, Longevity, and Enlightenment.* Roslindale: YMAA Publication Center, 1989.

Kaptchuk, Ted. *The Web That Has No Weaver: Understanding Chinese Medicine. 2nd ed.* New York: McGraw Hill, 2000.

Liangyue, Deng, and Cheng Xinnong. *Chinese Acupuncture and Moxibustion.* Beijing: Foreign Language, 1987.

Ni, Maoshing, and Cathy McNease. *The Tao of Nutrition.* Santa Monica: Seven Star Communication, 1987.

Veith, Ilza. *The Yellow Emperor's Classic of Medicine.* California: University of California Press, 2002.

Pitchford, Paul. *Healing with Whole Foods: Asian Traditions and Modern Nutrition. 3rd ed.* Berkley: North Atlantic Books, 2002.

Zhang, Ping. *A Comprehensive Handbook for Traditional Chinese Medicine Facial Rejuvenation.* Port Washington: Nefeli Corp., 2007.

Index

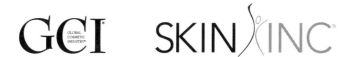

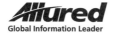